W9-CJL-387

Restoring Quality
Health Care

Restoring Quality Health Care

A Six-Point Plan for Comprehensive Reform at Lower Cost

Scott W. Atlas, MD

FARMINGDALE
PUBLIC
LIBRARY

HOOVER INSTITUTION PRESS

STANFORD UNIVERSITY | STANFORD, CALIFORNIA

www.hoover.org

Hoover Institution Press Publication No. 668

Hoover Institution at Leland Stanford Junior University,
Stanford, California 94305-6003

First printing 2016
22   21   20   19   18   17   16   8   7   6   5   4   3   2   1

Manufactured in the United States of America

The paper used in this publication meets the minimum Requirements of the American National Standard for Information Sciences—Permanence of Paper for Printed Library Materials, ANSI/NISO Z39.48-1992. ∞

Cataloging-in-Publication Data is available from the Library of Congress.
ISBN: 978-0-8179-1944-3 (cloth : alk. paper)
ISBN: 978-0-8179-1946-7 (epub)
ISBN: 978-0-8179-1947-4 (mobi)
ISBN: 978-0-8179-1948-1 (PDF)

Contents

List of Figures and Tables

Figures

Tables

Acknowledgments

My sincere thanks go to many of my colleagues and friends, especially John Cogan and Alvin Rabushka, for their helpful discussions and insights.

Introduction

The Affordable Care Act (ACA), frequently referred to as Obama-care, has pushed health care in the United States onto a drastically different, far more government-dominated pathway. Massive expansion of failing entitlement programs, huge new tax burdens, and unprecedented regulatory authority of the federal government over health insurance and the health care industry are now in place. These changes were instituted while ignoring, indeed even doubling down on, the fundamental problems with the existing system—the perverse incentives that have caused runaway costs and excluded millions of Americans from accessing the world's best medical care. Simultaneously and with remarkable irony, those countries with the longest experience under government-centralized health systems, including Sweden, the United Kingdom, and others, are increasingly footing the bill to shift patients toward private clinics and outside doctors to remedy their scandalous waits, poor quality, and escalating costs.

Time is of the essence. Years after the initial rollout of the ACA, the American people, the health care industry, and the courts still struggle to navigate the law. Under the new regulatory environment, consolidation within virtually all of the important sectors of health care, including hospitals and physician practices, pharmaceutical companies, and insurers, has accelerated. This is harmful to patients. Further implementation of the ACA will undoubtedly reverse the superior access and outstanding quality of care that distinguish American health care from the centralized systems that are failing the world over. Meanwhile, America's aging population will increasingly require medical care at an unprecedented level. To meet these demands, technological advances in our emerging era of clinically relevant molecular biology offer great promise for new treatments and breakthrough cures. Yet the current trajectory of the health system, particularly under Obamacare, threatens both the sustainability of the system and the essential climate for the innovation necessary to reach these potentials.

As the ACA proceeds to erode the positives of US health care without repairing the system's most important flaws, it is time for a fundamentally different approach to improving America's health system. Instead of framing health reform with the traditional trade-off, that is, "take away benefits, or raise taxes," my plan centers on a completely different paradigm—restoring the appropriate incentives in order to increase the quality of health care and simultaneously reduce its costs. To accomplish that goal, I propose a six-point, strategic, incentive-based reform plan for US health care. The foundation of my plan centers on highly incentivized, lower-cost catastrophic coverage and universal, significantly expanded health savings accounts (HSAs). The plan transforms the US health care system by instilling market-based competition and empowering consumers while reducing the federal government's authority over health care. It restores the originally intended purpose of health insurance—to protect against the risk of significant and unexpected health care costs. Using specific incentives and detailed proposals, the plan enhances the availability and affordability of twenty-first-century medical care and ensures continued health care innovation. Once this plan is fully implemented, conservative estimates indicate that private national health expenditures will decrease by roughly $2.75 trillion over the decade, federal government health expenditures will decrease by approximately $1.5 trillion over the decade, and access to high-quality health care will significantly improve. These savings will promote increased economic activity into other areas of the US economy. And perhaps most importantly, the health reforms in this plan reflect the key principles held by the American people about what they value and expect from health care in terms of access, choice, and quality.

Before I address the rationale for the proposed reforms necessary to achieve the above goals, we need to understand clearly the current state of US health care. This book will first examine the status of US health care, particularly in light of the ACA, and then delineate key reforms to meet the significant health care challenges facing the nation. Six major reforms are then described in detail, each with its underlying rationale, as follows: (1) expand affordable private insurance; (2) establish and liberalize universal HSAs to leverage consumer power; (3) instill appropriate incentives with rational tax treatment of health spending; (4) modernize Medicare for the twenty-first century as the population ages; (5) overhaul Medicaid to eliminate the two-tiered health system for poor Americans; and (6) strategically enhance the supply of medical care while ensuring innovation.

CHAPTER ONE

US Health Care Today:
Setting the Record Straight

America is facing its greatest health care challenges in history. Unprecedented demand for medical care is a certainty. According to the Department of Health and Human Services' Administration on Aging and US Census Bureau statistics, the number of Americans sixty-five and older has increased by a full six million in the past decade alone, to more than 13 percent of the overall population, while those age eighty-five and older have increased by a factor of ten from the 1950s to today's six million (Figure 1.1).

Older people tend to have the most disabling diseases, including heart disease, cancer, stroke, and dementia—the diseases that depend most on specialists and complex technology for diagnosis and treatment. Simultaneously, obesity, America's most serious health problem, has increased to crisis levels, already affecting more adults and children in the United States than in any other nation (Figure 1.2); given the known lag time for such risk factors to impact health, the next decades promise to reveal obesity's massive cumulative health and economic harms.

These daunting demographic realities combine with serious fiscal challenges in US health care that promise to worsen over the near future in the absence of change. America's national health expenditures now total more than $3.1 trillion per year, or more than 17.4 percent of gross domestic product (GDP), and they are projected to reach 19.6 percent of GDP by 2024.[1] Medicaid, originally covering 250,000 beneficiaries, has expanded to cover more than seventy million people[2] at a cost of $500 billion per year. Medicare spent less than $1 billion in its first year, but today it spends more than $260 billion annually on hospital benefits alone and $615 billion in total. With the aging of the baby boomer generation,

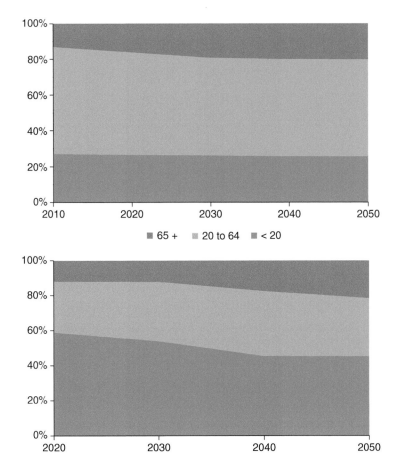

FIGURE 1.1. (*top*) Relative Age Distribution of Total US Population, 2010–2050; (*bottom*) Relative Age Distribution of Senior US Population, 2020–2050.
The population of seniors is rapidly growing. For those over sixty-five years of age, the proportions of seniors over seventy-five and over eighty-five are rapidly growing.
Source: US Census Bureau, "The Next Four Decades: The Older Population in the United States: 2010 to 2050" (based on 2008 data), https://www.census.gov/prod/2010pubs/p25-1138.pdf.

the program's costs in its current form appear unsustainable when one understands that in 1965, at the start of Medicare, workers paying taxes for the program numbered 4.6 per beneficiary, whereas that number will decline to 2.3 in 2030[3] (Figure 1.3).

The 2014 annual Medicare trustees report projects that the Hospitalization Insurance trust fund will face depletion in 2030.[4]

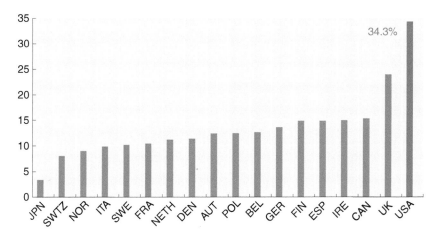

FIGURE 1.2. Obese Population (BMI > 30 Percent), Aged Fifteen and Above, Percentage of Population.
Prevalence of obesity (body mass index [BMI] of 30 percent or more) in United States and selected nations in the Organisation for Economic Co-operation and Development (OECD). The United States has more obese people than any other nation.
Source: Organisation for Economic Co-operation and Development, *OECD Fact Book 2010* (Paris, France: OECD, 2010), http://www.oecd-ilibrary.org/economics/oecd-factbook-2010_factbook -2010-en.

Regardless of trust fund depletion, Medicare and Medicaid must compete with other spending in the federal budget. With the current system, and barring new taxes and benefit cuts, federal expenditures for health care and social security are projected to consume all federal revenues by 2049, eliminating the capacity for national defense, interest on the debt, or any other domestic program.[5]

At the same time, we have entered an extraordinary era in medical diagnosis and therapy. Innovative applications of molecular biology, advanced medical technologies, new drug discoveries, and minimally invasive treatments promise earlier diagnoses and safer, more effective cures. The possibilities of improving health through medical advances have never been greater.

Before we consider reforms designed to reach the promise of twenty-first-century health care for all Americans, we need to understand the state of US health care prior to the Affordable Care Act. Whether defined by preventive screening tests;[6] waiting times for diagnosis or specialist appointments;[7] access to treatment for the

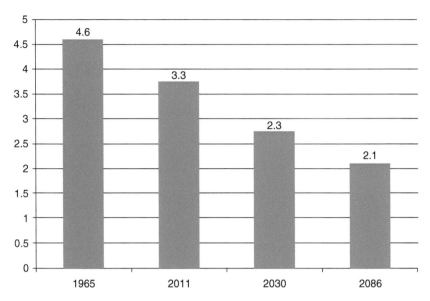

FIGURE 1.3. Workers Funding Medicare per Medicare Beneficiary, Historical and Projections.
The number of workers per beneficiary supporting Medicare is far less than at the beginning of the program and is rapidly declining.
Source: Centers for Medicare and Medicaid Services, Office of the Actuary, 2014 Annual "Report of the Boards of Trustees of the Federal Hospital Insurance and Federal Supplementary Medical Insurance Trust Funds," July 2014, https://www.cms.gov/research-statistics-data-and-systems/statistics-trends-and-reports/reportstrustfunds/downloads/tr2014.pdf.

major chronic diseases;[8] timeliness of biopsies for cancer;[9] waits for life-saving and life-changing surgeries;[10] or availability of safer medical technology[11] and the newest drugs[12] that save lives, Americans enjoyed unrivaled access to care.[13] And, just as important, the objective data from the world's leading medical journals prove that American medical care already delivered exceptional results for virtually all of the most serious diseases.[14] Those results include superior survival for major and rare cancers,[15] better outcomes from heart disease and stroke treatment,[16] and more successful treatment of chronic diseases such as hypertension and diabetes[17] than in those countries with centralized health systems heavily controlled by governments. The inescapable conclusion on the basis of the facts is that both quality of medical care and the access to it have been superior in the United States as compared with those nationalized systems heralded as models for change by ACA supporters (Figures 1.4 and 1.5).

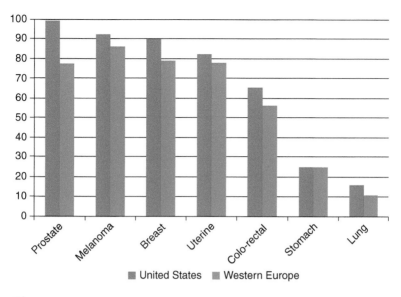

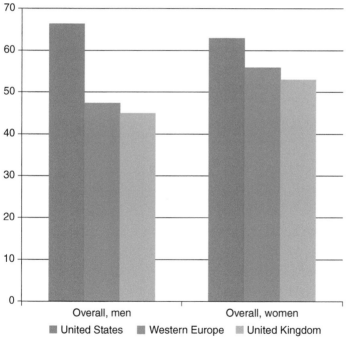

FIGURE 1.4. Five-Year Cancer Survival Rates (%).
(*top*) A comparison of five-year survival rate, United States versus western Europe, 2000–2002, seven common cancers. The United States has superior survival rates from all common cancers compared to western European nations. (*bottom*) Comparison of five-year survival rates for men and women, United States versus western European nations. Note a statistically significant increased survival rate for American men and women compared to the average western European nations and even more advantage over the United Kingdom.
Source: A. Verdecchia et al., "Recent Cancer Survival in Europe: A 2000–02 Period Analysis of EUROCARE-4 Data," *Lancet Oncology* 8 (2007): 784–96.

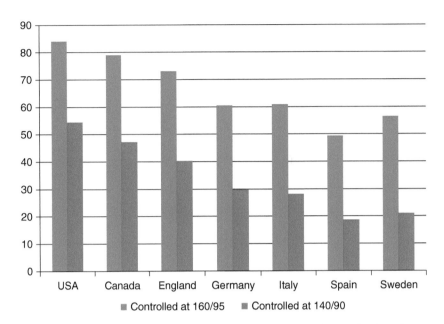

FIGURE 1.5. Successful Control of High Blood Pressure, Percentage of Treated Patients by Country, Ages Thirty-Five to Sixty-Four Years.
The United States has more effective medical care for high blood pressure compared to other developed countries, including those held as models for the ACA.
Source: From K. Wolf-Maier et al., "Hypertension Treatment and Control in Five European Countries, Canada, and the United States," *Hypertension* 43 (2004): 10–17.

Partly based on now-discredited studies alleging the poor quality of America's health care,[18] the ACA was enacted. Its two core elements, a significant Medicaid expansion and subsidies for exchange-based private insurance, will each cost about $850 billion over the next decade.[19] Fundamentally, the ACA consists of a huge centralization of health care and health insurance to the federal government, driving government centralization of health insurance to unprecedented levels while dramatically pushing up private insurance premiums. During the first three quarters of 2014, 89 percent of the newly insured under Obamacare were enrollees into Medicaid, not private insurance.[20] Together with population aging, the Centers for Medicare and Medicaid Services (CMS) projects that the 107 million people under Medicaid or Medicare in 2013 will rapidly increase to 135 million just five years later, a growth rate tripling that of private insurance.[21] At the same time, we are witnessing increasing consolidation under Obamacare in several areas of health care, including insurers, doctors, hospitals, and pharmaceutical companies. This ongoing consolidation is going to reduce competition and therefore hurt consumers.

But the goals of health reform demand quite the opposite. Facts show that private insurance is superior to government insurance for both access and quality of medical care (see chapter 2). History shows that the best way to control prices is through competition for empowered, value-seeking consumers. Instead of shunting more people into insurance and care provided by the government, heavily subsidized by the government, or massively regulated by the government, reforms should focus on how to produce competition-driven markets that will deliver innovation and cost savings, thereby maximizing the availability and affordability of the best care for everyone. The key is to move away from centralized models based on misguided incentives necessitating more and more taxation to one of individual empowerment with personal responsibility.

CHAPTER TWO

Reform #1:
Expand Affordable Private Insurance

Principal Features of Reform #1: Expand Affordable Private Insurance

- Permit all insurers (including all companies available on any state or federal exchanges) to offer true high-deductible, limited-mandate catastrophic coverage (LMCC) plans to all citizens, covering hospitalizations, outpatient visits, diagnostic tests, prescription drugs, and mental health.
- Transfer ownership of coverage to the individual so that it is portable; employer still available for sign up and automation of payments
- Permit insurers to eliminate Obamacare's 3:1 age-based premiums
- Permit insurers to risk-adjust premiums for obesity, as is already allowed for smoking.
- Eliminate the health insurance premium excise tax.

The Importance of Private Health Insurance

Broad access to doctors and hospitals comes with private insurance, not government insurance. The harsh reality awaiting low-income Americans is that most doctors already refuse to take new Medicaid patients because of government-defined low reimbursements, numbers that dwarf by eight to ten times the percentage that refuse to take new private insurance patients.[1] According to a 2014 Merritt Hawkins report, 55 percent of doctors in major metropolitan areas refuse to take new Medicaid patients.[2] The Department of Health and Human Services reported in December 2014 that even of those managed care providers signed by contract and on state lists to provide care to Medicaid enrollees, 51 percent were not available to new Medicaid patients.[3]

Like Medicaid, a superficial look at Medicare appears satisfactory to most of its beneficiaries, but on scrutiny we see a different scenario unfolding today. While the population ages into Medicare eligibility, a growing proportion of doctors do not accept Medicare patients. According to the Medicare Payment Advisory Commission, 29 percent of Medicare beneficiaries who were looking for a primary care doctor back in 2008 already had a problem finding one.[4] In 2012 alone, CMS reported that almost ten thousand doctors opted out of Medicare, nearly tripling from 2009; according to the Texas Medical Association, the number of Texas physicians accepting Medicare patients dropped to 58 percent in 2012. In a 2014 physician survey, about one-quarter of doctors no longer see Medicare patients or limit the number they see; in primary care, 34 percent refuse Medicare patients.[5] The percentage of doctors who closed their practices to Medicare or Medicaid by 2012 had increased by 47 percent since 2008.[6]

Beyond access to care, the quality of medical care is also superior with private insurance. For those with private insurance, that quality includes fewer in-hospital deaths, fewer complications from surgery, longer survival after treatment, and shorter hospital stays than similar patients with government insurance.[7] Restricted access to important drugs, specialists, and technology under government insurance most likely account for these differences.

The Harmful Impact of the ACA on Private Insurance

Affordable private insurance options have clearly not been improved by the ACA. As a direct result of the ACA's new regulations on pricing and its new mandates on coverage, the law has already forced more than five million Americans off of their existing private health plans. The Congressional Budget Office (CBO) projects that a stunning ten million Americans will be forced off their chosen employer-based health insurance by 2021—a tenfold increase in the number that was initially projected back in 2011.[8] Meanwhile, private insurance premiums have greatly increased under Obamacare and are projected to skyrocket in 2016, in some cases increasing by 30 percent to 50 percent and more. The shift into government insurance itself also increases private insurance premiums. Because government reimbursement for health care is often below cost, costs are shifted back to private carriers, pushing up premiums. In some calculations, the underpayment by government insurance adds $1,800 per year to every family of four with private insurance.[9] Nationally, the gap between private insurance payment and government underpayment has become the widest in twenty years, doubling since the initiation of Obamacare, according to a 2014 study by Avalere Health.[10] Even more ominous, consolidation among the five big private insurers has accelerated, a trend that most analysts believe will raise premiums for individuals and small businesses. This rise will impact not only the individual but also taxpayers, because taxpayers subsidize those increasing premiums under Obamacare.

Choices of private insurance and covered providers under them are dwindling as well, despite the theory that the law would increase insurance choices and competition. According to a December 2014 study,[11] the exchanges offer 21 percent fewer plans than the pre-Obamacare individual market, with a decrease to 310 nationally in 2015 compared to 395 insurers in the individual market in 2013, the last year before this implementation of Obamacare.

For middle-income Americans dependent on subsidized private insurance through government exchanges, Obamacare is also eliminating access to many of the best specialists and best hospitals. McKinsey reported that 68 percent of those policies cover only narrow or very narrow provider networks, double that of the previous year.[12] The majority of America's best hospitals in the National Comprehensive Cancer Network are not covered in most of their states' exchange plans. And as of late 2014, we are experiencing a severe shortage of the specialists essential to diagnose and treat stroke, one of the most disabling and lethal diseases in the United

States (in some cities, the number is actually down to zero) under Obamacare insurance plans.[13] The narrow network strategy is hitting even more Americans in 2015, as Obamacare exchange plans restrict access to doctors and hospitals far more than insurance bought off exchanges, in an attempt to quell insurance premium increases caused by the law itself.[14]

Keys to Expanding Affordable Private Insurance

Fundamental change to private insurance is vital to leveraging consumer power and expanding health care access for everyone. The ACA has made private insurance less affordable and pushed health insurance reform in the wrong direction. It has furthered the erroneous view that insurance should subsidize the entire gamut of medical services, including routine medical care. When that inappropriate function of insurance is combined with the cloak of secrecy shielding health care prices and provider qualifications, consumers have neither an incentive nor the necessary means to invoke value into health care decisions.

On the other hand, high deductibles with catastrophic coverage would restore the essential purpose of insurance—to reduce the risk of incurring large and unanticipated medical expenses. Because they would pay for most medical care directly, consumers would have the incentive to choose wisely. Provider prices would consequently become more visible and align with what consumers value, rather than being set artificially or by government decree.

The behavior of American consumers counters the ACA's approach to insurance reform and validates the argument that higher-deductible coverage both generates more affordable insurance and reduces health spending. In the decade since the tracking of this type of coverage, consumers have increasingly selected high-deductible plans (Figure 2.1), and among those enrollees, a shift toward higher deductibles has continued (Figures 2.2 and 2.3).[15] Consumer spending is significantly reduced for those in high-deductible plans,[16] without any consequent increases in emergency room visits

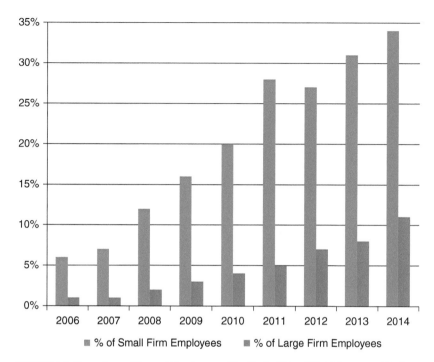

FIGURE 2.1. Percentage of Covered Employees with a Deductible of $2,000 or more, Single Coverage, by Firm Size and Year.
Consumers have increasingly chosen high-deductible coverage.
Source: Data compiled from Employer Annual Health Benefits surveys, Kaiser Family Foundation, http://kff.org/health-costs/report/employer-health-benefits-annual-survey-archives.

or hospitalizations and without the hypothesized harmful impact on low-income families or the chronically ill.[17] Health spending reductions averaged 15 percent annually, and the savings increased with the level of the deductible and when paired with HSAs. More than one-third of the savings by enrollees resulted from lower costs per health care utilization,[18] that is, value-based decision making by consumers. Additional evidence from studies of consumers' use of magnetic resonance imaging[19] and outpatient surgery[20] shows that introducing price transparency and defined-contribution benefits further encourages price comparisons by patients. While especially relevant to patients using high-deductible plans with HSAs, these reforms would reduce expenditures by all health care consumers.

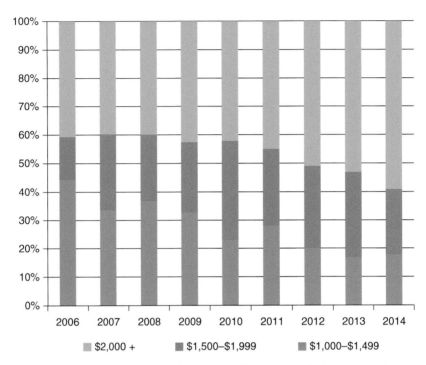

FIGURE 2.2. Deductible Distribution in High-Deductible Plans with Savings Account Options, by Year.
Among those enrolled into high-deductible coverage, consumers have shifted to higher deductibles.
Source: Data compiled from Employer Annual Health Benefits surveys, Kaiser Family Foundation, http://kff.org/health-costs/report/employer-health-benefits-annual-survey-archives.

Affordable private insurance, specifically with high deductibles and HSAs, should be a principal focus of health care reform (see chapter 3) in order to both improve benefits and reduce costs. To expand affordable private insurance options, we need to reduce onerous regulations on insurance, many of which have specifically harmed high-deductible plans. While consumers are still increasingly opting for plans with deductibles greater than $2,000, the growth rates have slowed compared to the growth before ACA mandates and restrictions (Figure 2.4). In addition, the premiums of high-deductible plans are accelerating faster after the passage of the ACA than any other coverage[21] (Figures 2.5 and 2.6), although they remain less costly than other types of coverage. We cannot be certain whether these changes are entirely caused

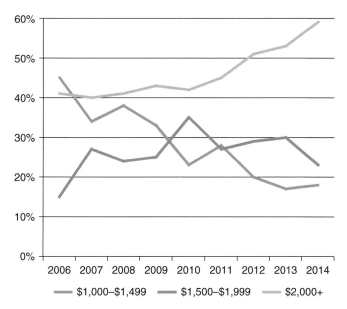

FIGURE 2.3. Trends in Deductible Distribution in High-Deductible Plans with Savings Account Options.
The shift of enrollment into higher deductibles for enrollees in high-deductible plans with associated savings accounts comes at the expense of the low-deductible range.
Source: Data compiled from Employer Annual Health Benefits surveys, Kaiser Family Foundation, http://kff.org/health-costs/report/employer-health-benefits-annual-survey-archives.

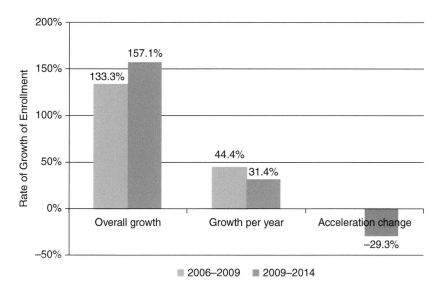

FIGURE 2.4. Enrollment Rate of Growth, Deductible of $2,000+, Single Coverage, All Firms, Before vs. After Passage of ACA.
The growth rates of enrollment into high-deductible plans have decelerated since the passage of the ACA.
Source: Data compiled from Employer Annual Health Benefits surveys, Kaiser Family Foundation, http://kff.org/health-costs/report/employer-health-benefits-annual-survey-archives.

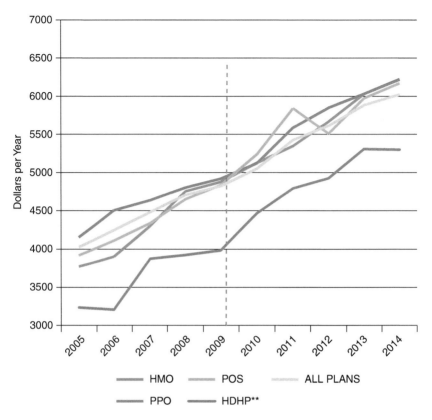

FIGURE 2.5. Premiums by Plan Type, Before vs. After Passage of ACA.
The annual premiums for all types of insurance coverage have increased over the past decade (vertical line indicates passage of ACA).
Notes: HMO, health maintenance organization; *PPO*, preferred provider organization; *POS*, point of service; *HDHP*, high-deductible health plan. Premiums include both employee and employer payments; **HDHP includes high-deductible plans offered with either a health reimbursement arrangement or HSA.
Source: Data compiled from Employer Annual Health Benefits surveys, Kaiser Family Foundation, http://kff.org/health-costs/report/employer-health-benefits-annual-survey-archives.

by Obamacare's regulations, such as limits on deductibles, but clearly health system reforms should not selectively make these plans less affordable for consumers. Restoring the choice of LMCC with truly high deductibles would add the more affordable coverage that many consumers value.

We should eliminate unnecessary coverage mandates that have ballooned under the ACA. Let's strip back many of Obamacare's so-called minimum essential benefits that have increased premi-

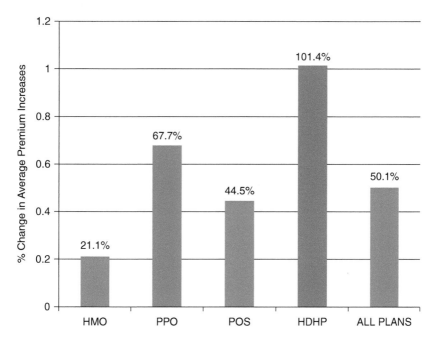

FIGURE 2.6. Acceleration of High-Deductible Health Plan Premium Increases (%) Before (2005-2009) vs. After (2009-2014) Passage of ACA.
Although all types of insurance plans have increased in price faster after the bill's passage compared to before the bill's passage, Obamacare regulations have accelerated the increase in premiums of high-deductible plans more than any other type of coverage.
Notes: HMO, health maintenance organization; *PPO*, preferred provider organization; *POS*, point of service; *HDHP*, high-deductible health plan. The high-deductible plans include those offered with either a health reimbursement arrangement or HSA; premiums include both employee and employer payments.
Source: Data compiled from Employer Annual Health Benefits surveys, Kaiser Family Foundation, http://kff.org/health-costs/report/employer-health-benefits-annual-survey-archives.

ums by almost 10 percent[22] and eliminate most of the more than 2,270 state mandates[23] requiring coverage for everything from acupuncture to marriage therapy. We should remove archaic obstacles to competition, including barriers to out-of-state insurance purchases. To eliminate unfair cost shifts imposed by the ACA that raised premiums for younger, healthier enrollees by 19 percent to 35 percent,[24] we should remove the 3:1 ACA dictate on actuarial regulations for age-rated premiums. Finally, we should repeal the ACA's new annual health insurance providers fee ($11.3 billion in 2015) that insurers pass on to enrollees through increased premiums, according to the CBO.[25] The ACA imposed this new sales tax on health insurance beginning in 2014, and the Joint Committee on Taxation (JCT) estimated that the tax burden will exceed $100 billion over its first decade and raise consumers' premiums by up to 3.7 percent per year. This specific tax will increase insurance costs by thousands of dollars over the decade for individuals, families, businesses, and even the beneficiaries of the government's own insurance programs—both Medicare and Medicaid.[26]

In addition, health insurance reform is a powerful opportunity to incentivize healthy lifestyles. Two behaviors deserve special consideration. Cigarette smoking and obesity are the two most important lifestyle behaviors, both proved to increase the risk for highly morbid chronic disease and worsen outcomes from those diseases, regardless of health care quality. Smoking causes $193 billion in direct health care expenditures and productivity losses each year, according to the Centers for Disease Control.[27] Extra medical care for obesity comprises up to 10 percent of total US health care costs.[28] Because of obesity's high prevalence and its association with multiple chronic diseases, worse treatment results, and more complications from even the best care, the annual US societal costs of obesity exceed $215 billion.[29] While smoking has declined, the burden of obesity to the US health care system and to taxpayers has increased to crisis levels. This situation will only increase over the coming decades, given that diseases from these risk factors typically show a lag time of twenty to twenty-five years. Even without a reduction, some of the costs could be alleviated. Eric Finkelstein of Duke University has projected that *"keeping obesity rates level could yield a savings of nearly $550 billion in medical expenditures over the next two decades."*[30] Health care reform in the United States urgently needs to embrace a new era of personal responsibility, and obesity, today's most serious public health problem of American society because of both costs and its damage to people's health, should be the highest priority.

Just as in other insurance, premiums that reflect the higher risk of disease and more frequent use of medical care as a consequence of voluntary, high-risk behavior are sensible, especially because three-fourths of health insurance claims may result from lifestyle choices.[31] Life insurance premiums are markedly higher for dangerous behavior such as smoking. Risky driving is a key factor in determining automobile insurance rates. Obesity and smoking are high-risk lifestyles, both of which are major drivers of health expense with well-known health hazards. A 1998 study showed that claims of individuals with a high body mass index (BMI) cost $3,537 (2015 dollars) more per year than claims of individuals with low BMI.[32] A 2012 study showed that annual medical costs for people who are obese were $1,429 higher in 2006 than those for people of normal weight; for Medicare patients, this difference was $1,723, with almost 40 percent the result of extra prescription drugs.[33] These numbers exceed the extra medical costs from smoking. A growing number of employers charge smokers higher insurance premiums. In the individual insurance market, the "obese BMI" category paid 22.6 percent more in premiums, and those with "overweight BMI" paid 12.8 percent more than "normal BMI" enrollees.[34] While acknowledging the complexity and limited knowledge about the influence of genetics on obesity development as well as the harmful health effects of obesity in any individual, actuarially based premium differences for obesity should be allowed in all health insurance plans.

CHAPTER THREE

Reform #2:
Establish and Liberalize Universal
Health Savings Accounts

Principal Features of Reform #2: Establish and Liberalize Universal Health Savings Accounts

---

- Open health savings accounts automatically for every citizen with a social security number (or at birth)
- Allow each individual to own a health savings account immediately
- Make all accounts fully portable, fully controlled by the individual
- Permit employer to still serve as center for sign ups and automated contributions to accounts
- Eliminate the requirement for specific deductibles in accompanying insurance coverage
- Allow higher contribution maximums to equal those of total annual out-of-pocket limits
- Permit broader uses for spending (health care products and services and use by family members)
- Ease limits on employer-provided financial incentives for wellness programs
- Allow tax-free rollovers of all health savings accounts to surviving family members

Independent health savings accounts allow individuals to set aside money tax free for *uncovered expenses*, including routine care. Both contributions and disbursements from the HSA are tax free as long as they are spent on health care. The tax incentives of HSAs are different from those in a policy of simply allowing a tax deduction for all out-of-pocket health spending. If all out-of-pocket spending was tax deductible, overall health spending would pay

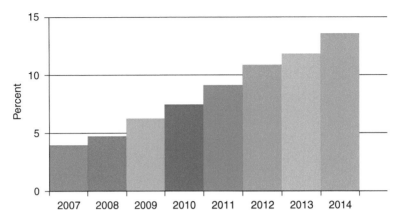

FIGURE 3.1. Enrollment into HSAs among Privately Insured, by Number of Accounts, for Adults under Sixty-Five, by Year.
Enrollment into HSAs has steadily increased since their introduction.
Source: CDC/National Health Care Surveys, National Health Interview Surveys, 2007–2014, Family Core component.

roughly seventy cents for each dollar of health care consumed. On the other hand, HSAs lower the cost of saving. They counter the tax bias against high-deductible plans in a unique way. Instead of simply introducing incentives that subsidize health care spending relative to other spending, they also incentivize saving.

Despite the ACA's restrictions, HSAs continue to grow. Indeed, by increasingly choosing HSAs when given the opportunity, American consumers are approving their value (Figure 3.1). HSAs have grown rapidly over the past decade, with a one-year jump of 29 percent as of the end of 2014, reaching a record high of 14.5 million as of mid-2015.[1] Nearly one-third of all employers (31 percent) now offer some type of HSA, up from just 4 percent in 2005. HSA account holders deposited $21 billion in 2014, and investment assets increased by 40 percent since the previous year, to an estimated $3.2 billion by year end. By the end of 2017, the HSA market will surpass $46 billion in assets held in almost twenty-five million accounts.

Beyond increasing the options for affordable private insurance, these consumer-empowering shifts pairing HSAs with high-deductible coverage reduces costs—the main goal of health system reforms in the first place. Adding HSAs to high-deductible plans provides more incentive to save than other arrangements; in Haviland's 2011 study, adding HSAs to high-deductible plans correlated to an increased savings of from 5.5 percent to 14.1 percent, or 50 percent to more than double the savings of high-deductible plans alone.[2] System-wide health expenditures would fall by an estimated $57 billion per year if only half of Americans with employer-sponsored insurance enrolled in plans combining HSAs with high deductibles.[3] Savings would increase further if deductibles were truly high, for example, $4,000–$5,000, and if these plans were freed from the added costly mandates of the ACA. Total savings from these reforms could approach $2 trillion over the decade.

The fundamental point is that HSAs, especially with high-deductible coverage, incentivize and leverage the power of consumers. This consumer power is crucial to making health care more affordable while maintaining health care excellence, access, and innovation. The issue is not whether these accounts are effective; it is how to maximize their adoption and eliminate the government rules that serve as obstacles to their use. The first step is to make HSAs available to all Americans, automatically opened for every citizen with a social security number or at birth. All HSAs should be owned by individuals, eliminating more restrictive variants that are tied to specific employers. We should immediately liberalize maximum contributions to the level of total annual out-of-pocket expenses under the ACA (for 2016, $6,850 for individuals and $13,700 for families), ease restrictions on their uses to extend to family members regardless of tax dependency, and allow rollovers to surviving family members. These changes would lower the after-tax burden to high spenders, that is, those with chronic diseases, making HSAs more useful to them. We should also eliminate the counterproductive requirement of owning coverage with government-specified deductibles in order to open an HSA. Removing this rule would introduce more consumer power and incentivize more families to save for out-of-pocket expenses.

TABLE 3.1. Key Changes in Proposed Health Savings Accounts

Topic	Current HSA	New HSA
General eligibility	Must meet many specific requirements (see below and text)	Universal for all citizens; automatically opened at birth
Insurance requirement to contribute to HSA	Government-specified high-deductible coverage	No specified deductible range of coverage
Limits on maximum contribution per year	$3,350 (individual) $6,750 (family)	$6,850 (individual) $13,700 (family)
Uses of HSA funds	Not for nonprescription drugs other than insulin; for self, spouse, and tax dependents only	Over-the-counter drugs are eligible without need for doctor's prescription; for self, spouse, children, parents, and siblings, regardless of tax dependency
Tax deductibility	Contributions and withdrawals deductible	Contributions and withdrawals deductible
Eligibility if enrolled in Medicaid	Not eligible without exemption	Eligible
Eligibility if enrolled in Medicare	Not eligible	Eligible
Eligibility if receiving Social Security	Not eligible	Eligible

Clearly, one could argue about the optimal maximum for HSAs or any other specific amount chosen in this reform package. It is important that we all recognize the purpose of health reforms—good health. HSAs are one important vehicle to achieve that ultimate goal. The differences between current regulations on HSAs and the proposed new rules for HSAs are summarized in Table 3.1 (also see "Key Questions and Answers on the Atlas Plan").

A growing number of employers are charging smokers higher insurance premiums while also offering wellness programs and medical screenings for risk factors, including such tests as blood pressure, body mass index, and cholesterol. In 2015, 96.7 percent of employers offered lifestyle programs,[4] increasing from 73 percent

TABLE 3.1. (continued)

Topic	Current HSA	New HSA
Special Medicare Advantage medical savings accounts (MSAs)	List of restrictions limiting contribution levels, contribution sources, others	Full conversion to standard HSA without any special limits or restrictions
Penalty for ineligible withdrawals	20 percent penalty (plus taxation)	50 percent penalty (plus taxation)
Use for insurance premiums (seniors only)	At age sixty-five, can reimburse yourself for the money that Social Security withholds from your benefits to pay Medicare Part B (which will be $104.90 per month for most people in 2015), and you can make tax-free HSA withdrawals to pay Medicare Part D and Medicare Advantage premiums (but not Medigap premiums)	Allowed for all premiums only if coverage is limited-mandate catastrophic plan
Seniors and ineligible withdrawals	After sixty-five, no penalty (just taxation)	After seventy (new Medicare eligibility age), 20 percent penalty (plus taxation)
Transfers into HSAs from retirement accounts	Not allowed	Allowed without penalty for seniors
Tax treatment to beneficiary on death of HSA holder	If spouse, tax-free rollover into HSA; otherwise, taxable income	If spouse or other family member, tax-free rollover into HSA

in 2011 and 57 percent in 2009. More than one-third of firms with wellness programs include financial incentives to participants, including lower insurance premiums, reduced cost sharing, and higher employer contributions to individual HSAs.[5] Consumers have demonstrated the efficacy of smoking cessation and obesity interventions, including cash financial incentives. Significant gains in productivity, marked reductions in health claims, improvement of chronic illnesses, and major cost savings have resulted and have benefited both participant employees and their employers.[6] Medical costs and absentee day costs fall by about three to six dollars for every dollar spent on wellness programs.[7] The ACA limits the financial incentives from employers, including cash deposits into employee HSAs, to 30 percent of the cost of that employee's health coverage—we should eliminate this unnecessary, arbitrary limit. Abolishing that limit would expand these powerful motivators for employees, encouraging employees to participate in more wellness programs already proved to improve health and reduce health costs.

CHAPTER FOUR

Reform #3:
Instill Appropriate Incentives
with Rational Tax Treatment
of Health Spending

Principal Features of Reform #3: Instill Appropriate Incentives
with Rational Tax Treatment of Health Spending

- Make tax treatment of health expenses universal, that is, equal for all, whether individual, self-employed, or employer-based
- Allow income tax and payroll tax exclusions for only two categories of expenses:
  - Limited-mandate catastrophic insurance premiums
  - HSA contributions for those with catastrophic insurance coverage
- Base income exclusion on new maximum HSA contribution (equivalent to the total annual out-of-pocket maximum, which approximately matches the 50th percentile of current employer health benefits)
- Index income exclusion increases to the Consumer Price Index for All Urban Consumers (CPI-U)

The income tax subsidy for unlimited health spending is one of the great mistakes of modern US tax policy. It creates harmful incentives for consumers that are counterproductive to competition and pricing, it replaces higher wages, and it is regressive, preferentially giving high-income earners more tax breaks.

Tax preferences for health care spending began as a somewhat unintended tax policy, as they arose from the fact that pension and health insurance fringe benefits provided by employers were not subject to wage controls imposed during World War II to maintain war production.[1] Later, employer payments for health benefits became deductible to employers and tax excluded to employees in the Internal Revenue Service tax code.[2] The current tax code sets no limits on this income exclusion, contrary to the original intent of Congress in 1954.[3]

The largest tax subsidy for private health insurance—the exclusion from income and payroll taxes of employer and employee contributions for employer-sponsored insurance—costs approximately $250 billion in lost federal tax revenue in 2013.[4] In addition, the federal tax deduction for health expenses (including premiums) exceeding 10 percent of the adjusted gross income is estimated to cost $12.4 billion in lost tax revenue in 2014.[5] The CBO projects that tax expenditure for employment-based insurance (including income and payroll taxes) will remain close to 1.5 percent of GDP during the coming decade.[6] The tax subsidy is highly preferential to individuals with higher incomes, that is, it is highly regressive. About 85 percent of the subsidy goes to individuals in the top one-half of the income distribution.[7] In addition, the tax exclusion distorts the labor market by limiting job mobility and strongly influencing retirement decisions.[8] Still, certain positives come from employer-sponsored insurance, such as risk pooling as well as the employees' opportunity to select insurance for more than one year at a time.

Beyond the numbers, the current tax exclusion creates perverse incentives. Indeed, the observation that "the tax subsidy is responsible for much of what is widely perceived as a health care crisis" may sound like it was written only recently, yet this statement dates back almost forty years.[9] The exclusion makes health spending seem less expensive than it is. The incentive to allocate more money for health care encourages more expensive insurance policies with more elaborate coverage as well as a higher demand for medical care regardless of cost. The current tax exclusion is preferential to insurance over out-of-pocket spending (as opposed to the incentive of HSAs, particularly as structured in this reform proposal). The distortion of health insurance to its now-dominant form that covers almost all billable services, including minor, fully predictable medical care, while minimizing direct payment by patients, is partly attributable to the tax preference. This preference has greatly increased the overall cost of health care.[10]

Changing the tax treatment of health spending is an important part of urgently needed health care reforms; unfortunately, comprehensive tax reform that would result in a broad-based, low-rate, simple system seems unlikely at this time. Removing the existing tax exclusion entirely would be problematic.[11] Serious repercussions could include a significant increase in the number of uninsured, an abrupt disruption of the labor market, and a dramatic increase in taxes.

Given those realities, the tax reform proposed herein eliminates the Obamacare excise tax and incorporates three main features: (1) universality regardless of the source of health benefits; (2) limits on the total allowed exclusion, and (3) new criteria on eligible spending for tax exclusion, limited only to HSA contributions and premium payments for LMCC. These tax reforms would reduce expenditures and encourage value-based insurance purchasing, that is, they would realign incentives in health insurance and health care markets to benefit consumers. Once the reforms are enacted, the increase in the individual's purchasing power for medical care more than compensates for the loss of certain tax subsidies for health care spending. Each reform is discussed in more detail below.

Universality

The current system is unfair and preferentially benefits higher-income earners who receive health benefits from employers. Current law permits families without employer-based health insurance to deduct medical expenses only if they itemize their deductions, a strategy chosen far more frequently by upper-income earners;

moreover, the deduction is limited to expenses that exceed 10 percent of adjusted gross income. To level the playing field, I propose that all citizens be allowed the same deductibility of health expenses if they purchase the basic LMCC. The proposed income exclusion for health spending will be applicable to all, regardless of employment or source of health benefits.

Total Allowable Exclusion Limit

The proposed allowable exclusion from income and payroll taxes is based on the maximum allowable HSA contribution ($6,850), roughly equal to the 50th percentile of current health benefits paid through employment.[12] For 2014, the estimated annual health insurance premium paid per worker equaled $6,025 for individual coverage; the average premium paid for high-deductible coverage equaled $5,280. Still, the term "high deductible" was defined as plans with annual deductibles only greater than or equal to $1,250 for an individual ($2,500 for a family); it also included coverage bloated by all of the ACA mandates and regulations. In the final year before ACA regulations, 2009, the average premium of high-deductible plans equaled 82.6 percent of the average cost of employer-provided health insurance, based on annual surveys of employer health benefits. Therefore, given other reforms in this six-point proposal that would further reduce the cost of true high-deductible coverage, the new exclusion should cover the entire cost of high-deductible plans plus significant deposits to HSAs.

The CBO and the JCT estimate that setting income exclusion limits on the basis of the 50th percentile for health insurance benefits paid by or through employers in 2015 (and indexed in subsequent years for inflation using the CPI-U), with the same limits for the deduction for health insurance available to self-employed people, would reduce deficits by $537 billion over the next decade.[13] This cap would have far greater impact on upper-income earners.[14] (Note, for contrast, that the Urban Institute estimated that capping the exclusion at the 75th percentile of total health benefit through employment would produce $264 billion in new income and pay-roll tax revenues over the coming decade.[15])

Eligible Spending for Income Exclusion

Current health spending eligible for tax exclusion is both unlimited in size (until the 2018 Obamacare "Cadillac tax" implementation [see the following paragraph for more on this tax]) and essentially unlimited in scope of eligible expenses. My proposal would add incentives for purchasing basic catastrophic coverage, beyond limiting the amount of the income exclusion and in addition to other incentives already described. Excludable health spending will apply only to two health expenses: (1) deposits to HSAs; and (2) premium payments for high-deductible, limited-mandate catastrophic coverage. It would be counterproductive to encourage the purchase of insurance bloated with expensive coverage requirements that minimize copays and effectively eliminate concern about prices of care. Added insurance coverage, including expensive "comprehensive" coverage, will always be available to those who wish to purchase it.

Note that my plan replaces the changes to the current tax exclusion under Obamacare set to begin in 2018. Under Obamacare, a new excise tax is set to be imposed on employment-based health benefits whose total value—including employers' and employees' tax-excluded contributions for insurance premiums and contributions made through health reimbursement accounts, flexible spending accounts, or HSAs for other health care costs—is greater than specified thresholds (subsequently to be indexed to the growth of the CPI-U). The JCT and the CBO project that those thresholds will be $10,200 for single coverage and $27,500 for family coverage in 2018. The excise tax (known as the "Cadillac tax") will equal 40 percent of the difference between the total value of tax-excluded contributions and the threshold. But designing a policy whereby a government imposes new taxes on products whose prices became unnecessarily high directly because of the government's policies is not only bad for consumers but frankly absurd. Moreover, the Cadillac tax is set to include contributions that employers and individuals make to HSAs toward the thresholds for invoking the 40 percent excise tax. This is a classic example of a misguided government intervention harming an excellent consumer-oriented program (HSAs and high-deductible plans), ironically penalizing individuals trying to lower their health expenses.

CHAPTER FIVE

Reform #4:
Modernize Medicare for
the Twenty-First Century

Principal Features of Reform #4: Modernize Medicare for the Twenty-First Century

- Introduce competitive bidding to add private insurance options for all Medicare enrollees

  - Define the benefit as premium support, calculated from a regional benchmark average price of three lowest-priced approved plans
  - Include the premium for LMCC high-deductible coverage as one of the three plans determining the benchmark average
  - Require all plans defining the calculated benchmark to include prescription drug benefits
  - Provide cash rebates to individual HSAs if the beneficiary chooses a plan with a premium less than benchmark; require payment from enrollees if premiums exceed benchmark

- Include catastrophic coverage in all plans eligible for Medicare program (that is, annual out-of-pocket limits)
- Combine old Parts A, B, and D to simplify deductibles, payments
- Establish expanded HSAs for all Medicare enrollees

  - Automatically open account for every Medicare enrollee; have limits and uses match other HSAs
  - Convert current HSA variants under Medicare to universal HSAs
  - Permit tax-free rollovers of all HSAs to surviving family

- Phase out taxpayer subsidies for high-income-earning seniors
- Modernize eligibility with gradual phase-in to age seventy
- Repeal the Independent Payment Advisory Board

Medicare is a tax expenditure targeted at the elderly who have already at least partially paid tax contributions over the years for their future health care insurance. Originally, Medicare was put forward as a safety net for protecting senior citizens from financial ruin by catastrophic illness. A key rationale for Medicare was that the program would enable seniors to avoid financial dependence, as evidenced by their lower incomes. This thinking ignored the fact that senior citizens had more substantial assets than younger adult populations during the years of the passage of the Medicare bill.[1] Even more ironic, original Medicare never had and, even today, traditional Medicare still does not include catastrophic insurance for asset protection.

Regardless of its origins, today's Medicare is highly fragmented, almost undecipherable in its complexity, flawed in its coverage, and inadequate in its benefits. After decades of coverage additions and patchwork remedies, today's Medicare is a confusing amalgam of four relatively separate insurance programs, each with complicated and diverse funding sources. Part A (hospital insurance) covers inpatient services, some home care, skilled nursing services, and hospice care. It is funded through the federal payroll tax by today's working population and employers. Most people do not pay a premium for Part A because they (or a spouse) have already paid via their payroll taxes while employed, although they do pay deductibles and copayments. Part B (medical insurance) covers doctor bills, outpatient treatment, screening and lab tests, and certain medical supplies, subject to deductibles and copayments. It is funded partly by beneficiaries via income-adjusted monthly premiums and partly by general tax revenues. Part C (Medicare Advantage, or MA) is a private insurance system that includes Part A and Part B benefits (i.e., it replaces Parts A and B, so-called traditional Medicare coverage), as well as some prescription drug coverage, for regional beneficiaries. As opposed to traditional Medicare, MA plans must have annual out-of-pocket limits (i.e., catastrophic coverage). In MA, Medicare contracts with private insurers to offer health services through a variety of provider networks, most commonly health maintenance organizations. MA is funded partly by member premiums and partly by capitated payments from taxpayer funds (note that since 2006, Medicare has paid plans under a bidding process, whereby Medicare receives bids from private insurers for coverage equal to Parts A and B and then pays the insurer for coverage relative to formulaic benchmarks by county or region). Part D (prescription drug coverage) is funded by income-adjusted enrollee premiums and taxpayer funds, as is Part B; copayments and deductibles vary by plan. In Part D, private insurance companies provide the coverage. Beneficiaries choose the drug plan and pay a monthly premium. In addition to this enormous programmatic complexity, Medicare administrators process nearly 4.9 million Medicare claims each business day, according to CMS. Unsurprisingly, the Medicare program is fraught with errors, fraud, and waste estimated by the Government Accountability Office to have totaled $60 billion in 2014.[2]

Medicare not only is a disjointed and antiquated system designed for decades long past; even more critical, it is in serious financial trouble. As noted in chapter 1, the Medicare trustees report projects that the Hospitalization Insurance fund will be depleted in 2030. Meanwhile, the population of seniors is dramatically expanding, and the taxpayer base financing the program is dramatically shrinking. In its first year, Medicare spent under $1 billion for 250,000 senior citizens, but in 2014 it spent over $615 billion for more than fifty-two million enrollees. Nearly four million Americans now reach age sixty-five every year. In 2050, the sixty-five-and-over population is projected to reach 83.7 million, almost double the 43.1 million in 2012. And the future health care needs for seniors have dramatically increased. The already high health expenses for a sixty-five-year-old (Figure 5.1) will triple by 2030.[3] Americans live 25 percent longer after age sixty-five now than in 1972,[4] with an average life expectancy of about eighty-five years, approximately five years longer than at the inception of

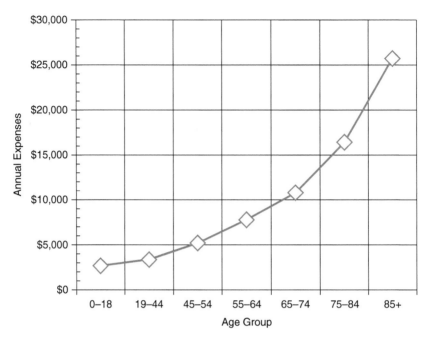

FIGURE 5.1. Per Capita Health Care Expenses, by Age, 2004.
Age is a clear predictor of health care utilization and health care costs per person.
Source: Centers for Medicare and Medicaid Services.

Medicare (Figure 5.2). Today's seniors need to save money for decades, not just years, of future health care.

Despite expanding needs from demographics, Obamacare imposed a new obstacle to health care access for seniors. Its Independent Payment Advisory Board (IPAB), a group of political appointees, is specifically given the task of formulaically reducing payments to doctors and hospitals. As Howard Dean, former chair of the Democratic National Committee, warned, "The IPAB is essentially a health-care rationing body. By setting doctor reimbursement rates for Medicare and determining which procedures and drugs will be covered and at what price, the IPAB will be able to stop certain treatments its members do not favor by simply setting rates to levels where no doctor or hospital will perform them."[5] The IPAB adds to Medicare's already significant access constraints; contrary to the

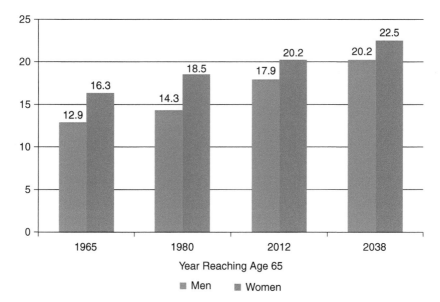

FIGURE 5.2. Additional Years of Life Expectancy in United States for Sixty-Five-Year-Olds, 1965–2038.
The additional life expectancy for those already reaching sixty-five years of age has increased greatly since 1965, when Medicare began.
Source: CDC/National Center for Health Statistics, *National Vital Statistics Reports* 62, no. 7 (January 2014).

administration's demonization of private insurers, *Medicare already ranks at the top of the charts for the highest rates of claim refusals— more than nearly all comparison private insurers every year.*[6]

Traditional Medicare often obstructs the delivery of health care and limits choices of doctors by virtue of its complex restrictions and rules about accepting "assignment" of Medicare insurance. "Assignment" means that a doctor has agreed to accept the Medicare-approved amount as full payment for services. Other doctors have not agreed to accept assignment, but they can choose to on a case-by-case basis. For these "non-participating" doctors, Medicare pays 5 percent less than their usual fees. Regardless of how much the health care provider charges non-Medicare patients for the same service, a Medicare patient cannot be charged more than 15 percent over the amount Medicare approves, that is, the "limiting charge." Doctors who formally "opt out" can charge patients whatever they want, but they must forgo filing Medicare claims for two years, and their Medicare-eligible patients must pay out of pocket to see them. By law, seniors are not allowed to use their Medicare benefits to pay doctors privately via their own arrangement.

The resulting trend is clear—doctors are increasingly refusing traditional Medicare and opting out of Medicare entirely. This trend promises to accelerate.[7] To prevent the escalation of two-tiered access to quality medical care, available only to affluent seniors, we need to empower all seniors to become value-seeking health care consumers. This empowerment also promises to be particularly effective for reducing inflated expenditures systemwide because seniors are the heaviest users of health care.

Seniors have shown the path toward Medicare reform—and that path is private insurance. In fact, more than 70 percent of Medicare beneficiaries already purchase private insurance to supplement or replace traditional Medicare.[8] About 23 percent of beneficiaries buy Medigap plans. These state-based private insurance plans that supplement nondrug Medicare benefits are available only to those enrolled in traditional Medicare (A and B) and not to MA enrollees. Voluntary enrollment in alternative Medicare Advantage private health plans, with the catastrophic coverage that is missing from traditional Medicare, has expanded to 31 percent of all Medicare beneficiaries, tripling since 2004 to 16.8 million in 2015.[9] Private prescription drug coverage in Part D, also with catastrophic caps, has also been highly favored by beneficiaries. Nevertheless, even in these private plans, Medicare ultimately defines the prices for medical care via complex and rather arbitrary capitated payments and other benchmarks,[10] thereby controlling access while, in some cases, wasting money.

Some elements of the fifty-year-old Federal Employees Health Benefits Program (FEHBP),[11] Congress' successful health insurance benefit program based on competition and consumer choice, serve as a model for reforming Medicare. In fact, the FEHBP served as the model for successful parts of current Medicare that rely on competition, that is, MA and Medicare Part D. Instead of government-directed traditional Medicare, the FEHBP contains almost three hundred plans from almost one hundred different companies that compete for business. The government provides money toward the premium of the plan chosen by the enrollee. Plan design, covered services, and costs emerge from competition and the value-seeking decisions of the individual consumer. In direct contrast to traditional Medicare, FEHBP's oversight agency, the Office of Personnel Management, does not establish payment rates to providers. Prior to Obamacare's mandates, each plan was free to offer benefits within very broad limits, including deductibles, covered services, limits on services, and copays. Other Medicare reform proposals, particularly the "Saving the American Dream" plan from Butler,[12] also serve as models for the reforms proposed herein.

Modernizing Medicare for the twenty-first century centers on a three-pronged strategy. This strategy will empower seniors to move to affordable private health insurance and HSAs, keys to improving benefits and reducing costs. The three elements of the strategy—a defined-contribution model, markedly expanded HSAs, and modernization of eligibility—are discussed in detail as follows.

Element #1: A Defined-Contribution Model

The first element of Medicare reform is implementing a defined-contribution model that offers private insurance options for beneficiaries with competition-based premiums and simplified benefits, as well as consumer incentives to seek value. The basic concept of this model is that the government would make a defined, fixed contribution, that is, a "premium support," to the private health plan of a Medicare enrollee's choice. Medicare will make market-based payments to competing insurance plans, not arbitrarily set prices and then pay health care providers. This way, the government's role changes from being a direct insurer to helping beneficiaries buy insurance. Similar to a number of previous reform proposals, the amount of the government's defined-contribution benefit will be based on the average of the three lowest-priced plans put forth to Medicare. This index group forming the calculated benchmark would include one limited-mandate high-deductible plan. All Medicare-eligible plans would be required to have annual out-of-pocket limits, that is, the catastrophic coverage that is missing from current traditional Medicare. All plans would also be required to offer prescription drug benefits.

If a beneficiary chooses a plan with a premium less than the benchmark, then a rebate payment of the entire difference would be made into that individual's HSA; if payment was due from the enrollee because of higher cost than the benchmark, the enrollee would be responsible. This would save more than the $15 billion per year the CBO estimates based on using higher benchmarks.[13] In this plan, the taxpayer premium subsidies for the highest-income earners would be lower but completely phased out at the highest levels. Medicare enrollees would be able to purchase more coverage by paying more in addition to the fixed government contribution.

Coverage would simplify the current separation of inpatient and outpatient expenses, unifying deductibles and payments fragmented into Medicare Part A and Part B. Ultimately, the goal is to eliminate the confusing and unnecessary separation of all inpatient and outpatient coverage, including MA plans and prescription drug coverage. In the long run, traditional Medicare will have been moved to private health insurance to improve access to doctors, hospitals, and modern medical technology and drugs; to improve benefits; and to reduce costs for all enrollees. For those over age thirty-five today, traditional Medicare will still remain an option; for those under age thirty-five, traditional Medicare coverage will no longer be provided.

Element #2: Expanded Eligibility and Uses of Health Savings Accounts

The second important element of modernized Medicare is new access to broadly expanded HSAs for all beneficiaries. Presently,

HSAs are quite limited in their allowed role for seniors. In fact, as noted earlier, the current laws prohibit Medicare enrollees from HSA eligibility. Seniors who have applied for or accepted Social Security cannot contribute to an HSA. Restricted accounts called "Medicare Advantage MSAs" are currently available but require enrollment in a high-deductible MA health plan. Among other restrictions (see "Key Questions and Answers on the Atlas Plan"), deposits into these MSAs are prohibited except from Medicare itself and are limited in amount to typically less than half of the required deductible of the accompanying coverage. On the death of the owner, HSAs are deemed taxable unless the beneficiary is the spouse.

Given that future health care needs for today's seniors now last decades, expanded HSAs will be of great importance to a modernized Medicare. HSA holders also participate more in wellness programs that focus on obesity and other major risks associated with chronic disease, increasingly relevant to senior care. New Medicare HSAs will be transformed into highly flexible vehicles for seniors to seek the best value for their health care spending (see "Key Questions and Answers on the Atlas Plan"). Under this plan, Medicare enrollees will automatically open HSAs if they had none before entering Medicare eligibility. Also under this plan, all Medicare enrollees will be fully eligible for HSAs regardless of enrollment into any specific coverage or program and without any specified level of deductible on insurance. The only requirement for making contributions to the HSA will be that the enrollee has catastrophic coverage. HSAs under new Medicare will have far higher maximum contribution limits (approximately double those for 2016), matching all other HSAs in the newly reformed system; likewise, they will have the same broadened uses of non-Medicare HSAs, including nonprescription medications and home health care devices. All current Medicare MSA limits and rules for uses will be updated to match universal HSA regulations, including removing the requirement to enroll in coverage with arbitrarily defined deductibles and eliminating Medicare MSA's restrictions on deposits. Because seniors typically incur greater health care costs, they will be allowed to roll over, tax free, money from retirement accounts into their HSAs. Seniors, their families, and their employers will all be allowed to contribute to the new HSAs up to the annual maximum. People will also be permitted to use their own HSA dollars for the health expenditures of their elderly parents regardless of tax dependency status. Even if Social Security benefits have begun, seniors will still be allowed to fund their HSAs. In new Medicare HSAs, a 20 percent penalty will be in place for nonqualified HSA withdrawals once the owner of the HSA becomes seventy years old. On the death of an enrollee, new Medicare HSA balances will be allowed to be rolled over to the tax-free HSA of the surviving spouse or other family members. This feature will also enhance HSA balances of younger family members and perpetuate increased consumer leverage on pricing.

Element #3: The Modernization of Eligibility

The third element of Medicare reform is the updating of eligibility from obsolete criteria of fifty years ago to reflect the demographics and health needs of today's seniors. The rationale to change these archaic eligibility criteria is straightforward. Modern medical care in the United States has increased life expectancy from birth by 1.6 years per decade for a half-century. Life expectancy from age sixty-five has increased about five years since program inception, equating to about one year longer from age sixty-five per decade that passes. Thus those individuals currently thirty-five years old will add another three years to their post-age-sixty-five life span. Moreover, older people now remain in the workforce longer. Retirement age has increased by five years since the early 1990s.[14] Under the proposed new Medicare, the age of eligibility would increase by two months per year until the individual reaches age seventy; after that, the eligibility age would be indexed to life expectancy. From CBO estimates, savings of about $65 billion over the decade would result from slowly phasing in this change.[15]

CHAPTER SIX

Reform #5:
Overhaul Medicaid
and Eliminate the Two-Tiered
System for Poor Americans

Principal Features of Reform #5: Overhaul Medicaid and
Eliminate the Two-Tiered System for Poor Americans

- Provide private insurance options for all Medicaid enrollees without
  need for special waivers

  - Permit all insurers, including all companies available on state
    and federal exchanges, to offer true high-deductible, LMCC
    plans (covering hospitalizations, outpatient visits, diagnostic
    tests, prescription drugs, and mental health) to the entire state
    population, including those eligible for Medicaid
  - Eliminate the requirement of special waivers for Medicaid
    enrollment into private insurance

- Establish and seed fund HSAs for all Medicaid enrollees

  - Open HSA automatically for every Medicaid enrollee and have
    limits and uses match other HSAs
  - Create new incentives for healthy behavior, which will save and
    protect growing financial assets
  - Ensure that seed funding goes directly into HSAs as part of
    federal contribution every year
  - Permit tax-free rollovers of all HSAs to surviving family members

- Change federal contribution to states for Medicaid to fixed
  amounts but with threshold-based incentives

  - Ensure that at least 50 percent of Medicaid enrollees are
    enrolled in LMCC plans
  - Ensure that at least 50 percent of Medicaid enrollees have at
    least partially funded HSAs

Medicaid is different from Medicare. Medicaid is generally a sub-sidy for the poor, paid by federal funds and state funds. Medic-aid is intended to help provide access to good medical care and improved health for those who cannot afford it. Instead of provid-ing a pathway to excellent health care for poor Americans, how-ever, Obamacare's expansion of Medicaid continues and even exacerbates their second-class health care status and does so at a cost of $500 billion per year to taxpayers, a cost that rises to $890 billion in 2024.[1] As an alternative, a few states have taken the lead within the confines of the ACA via special waivers to facilitate a transition into private coverage with better access to medical care. Arkansas and Iowa have received approval to use the "private option" in which Medicaid provides premium assistance to pur-chase private plans in lieu of direct Medicaid coverage.[2] In Arkan-sas, about 85 percent of Medicaid beneficiaries are now eligible for the private option, and as of January 1, 2015, Iowa has used it as an option for enrollees with income between 100 percent and 133 percent of the federal poverty level. In addition, Michigan and Indiana have added HSA options for Medicaid beneficiaries, and Arkansas has begun the approval process. Although these Medicaid pilot projects are still burdened with a mandated set of benefits and other regulations under the ACA, these states' efforts are steps in the right direction.

FIGURE 6.1. (*top, facing page*) **Percentage of Doctors* Accepting New Medicaid Patients, 2009 vs. 2013 Overall, Fifteen US Major Metropolitan Areas.** (*bottom, facing page*) **Percent-age of Medicaid-Contracted Providers Who Could Offer an Appointment to a New Medicaid Patient, by Type of Provider, 2014.**
Most doctors do not accept Medicaid patients, and the proportion of doctors who accept new Medicaid patients has been decreasing. Even of the doctors already contracted by Medicaid and listed as accepting patients, a large percentage do not accept new Medicaid patients. Obama-care has massively expanded Medicaid enrollment, but most enrollees will not be able to find doctors who will accept them as patients.
Note: *Includes cardiology, dermatology, obstetrics and gynecology, orthopedics, and family practice.
Sources: (*top*): Merritt Hawkins, "Physician Appointment Wait Times and Medicaid and Medicare Acceptance Rates, 2014 Annual Survey," http://www.merritthawkins.com/uploadedFiles /MerrittHawkins/Surveys/mha2014waitsurvPDF.pdf 2014; (*bottom*): Department of Health and Human Services, "Access to Care: Provider Availability in Medicaid Managed Care" Report OEI-02-13-00670 (December 2014), http://oig.hhs.gov/oei/reports/oei-02-13-00670.pdf.

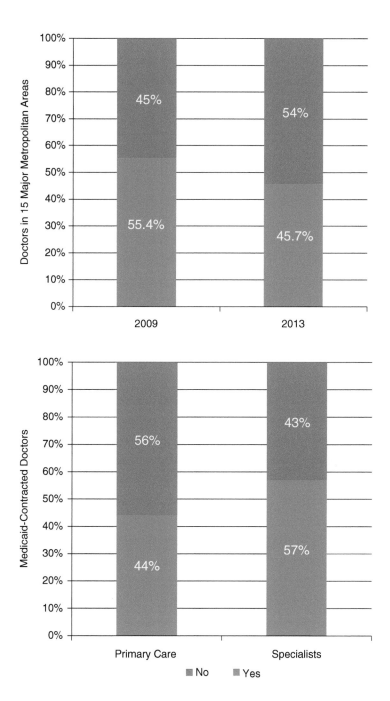

The time is long overdue for a more fundamental overhaul of Medicaid, with more aggressive reforms to truly modernize it into a program with improved benefits and ultimately reduced costs. Traditional Medicaid is essentially sham insurance that most doctors do not even accept (Figure 6.1).

My plan transforms Medicaid into a bridge program geared toward enrolling beneficiaries into affordable private insurance instead of a parallel second-class system funneling low-income families into substandard traditional Medicaid coverage. The plan establishes and seed funds HSAs, a vital component of empowering enrollees with the same control and incentives as all other Americans while instilling incentives for good health. These reforms would change the purpose and culture of Medicaid agency offices from running special government-administered Medicaid plans to establishing HSAs and finding private health plans for Medicaid beneficiaries.

The new Medicaid will have several features. First, new Medicaid will include a LMCC private insurance option for all enrollees, without any need for special waivers. Second, new Medicaid will establish and seed fund HSAs for the program's low-income American enrollees, in turn creating growing assets and incentivizing healthy lifestyles to protect those assets. To ensure the availability of the same health care to Medicaid enrollees as is available to Americans outside the program, federal funding will be available only to states that offer these same private coverage options to the entire state population, including Medicaid-eligible and non-eligible families; moreover, that funding will be contingent on meeting certain enrollment thresholds for Medicaid enrollees into LMCC private coverage and funding into HSAs. Funds will be allocated via fixed dollar amounts to states, but directly toward individual HSAs or insurance premium payments rather than into inefficient state bureaucracies. Ultimately, traditional Medicaid coverage will be eliminated over decades as new enrollees move toward private plans with HSAs.

The new Medicaid will financially empower low-income Americans to (1) purchase affordable, private insurance identical to what any American citizen could buy; and (2) fund HSAs that provide control and choice and, just as important, build assets worth protecting. These incentive-based Medicaid reforms would move Medicaid enrollees to private coverage, with equal access to doctors, specialists, treatments, and medical technology as the general population, eliminating the two-tiered health system that Obamacare furthers. It would give control of the health care dollar to low-income families to empower value seeking and foster provider competition for that money. Medicaid HSAs would provide new incentives for lower-income families to seek good health through wellness programs and healthy behavior in order to save and protect their new, growing financial assets.

Reform #6: Strategically Enhance the Supply of Medical Care While Ensuring Innovation

Principal Features of Reform #6: Strategically Enhance the Supply of Medical Care While Ensuring Innovation

- Stimulate and publicize private retail clinics staffed by nurse practitioners and physician assistants and minimize obstacles and unnecessary regulatory burdens
- Encourage streamlined training programs for physicians and abolish power of medical specialty societies and other administrative bodies that artificially restrict the supply of trained specialists and inhibit competition
- Loosen the scope of practice restraints on nurse practitioners and physician assistants
- Institute national physician licensing via state reciprocity
- Repeal innovation-limiting ACA taxes on medical devices and brand-name drugs
- Streamline the bureaucracy of the Food and Drug Administration (FDA) with regard to device and drug approvals
- Implement strategic immigration reforms to target high-skilled foreign workers and facilitate longer-term visas for highly educated immigrants

Challenges to health care access cannot be met without strategically modernizing the supply and delivery of medical care. Private sector clinics owned by pharmacies and staffed by nurse practitioners and physician assistants can provide routine primary care, including administering flu shots, monitoring blood pressure, conducting blood tests, and dispensing inexpensive drugs. In a 2011 review, researchers found that eleven medical conditions (outside of preventive care and immunizations) accounted for 88 percent of acute care visits to retail clinics; all the treatments involved relatively low medical costs.[1] Care initiated at retail clinics is 30–40 percent cheaper than similar care at physician offices and about 80 percent cheaper than at emergency departments.[2] Patients seek care at these clinics for several reasons, particularly convenience (that is, extended hours, no need for appointments, and convenient locations), low-cost services, short wait times, and transparent pricing;[3] they have generally reported high levels of satisfaction with their care. Accenture estimates that retail clinics can potentially save hundreds of millions of dollars per year while increasing neighborhood access to routine primary care.[4] While private ownership by stores or pharmacies is common, an emerging trend is for independent retail clinics to develop formal relationships with hospital systems or physician groups. The use of such clinics increased tenfold between 2007 and 2009[5] and continues to grow 15 percent annually. The percentage of large employers providing benefits covering retails clinics nearly doubled between 2008 and 2009. Nearly all accept private insurance (97 percent) and Medicare fee for service (93 percent),[6] but only 60 percent accepted traditional Medicaid.

The key to incentivizing the proliferation of these clinics may rest on eliminating government and special interest obstacles to their use. Retail clinics should not be held to higher standards or more burdensome documentation than other health care clinics. Credentialing requirements for insurance reimbursement should be simplified. In addition, states should follow the recommendations of the Institute of Medicine[7] and remove outmoded scope-of-practice limits and politically based practice restrictions on nurse practitioners and physician assistants, starting first with the dozen states categorized as having "restricted practice" regulations.

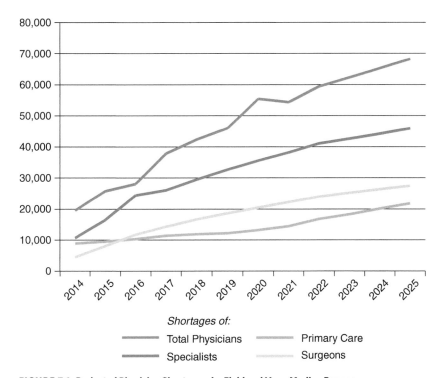

FIGURE 7.1. Projected Physician Shortages, by Field and Year, Median Ranges.
The projected shortages of specialists and surgeons exceed the projected shortage of primary care doctors.
Source: IHS Inc., "The Complexities of Physician Supply and Demand: Projections from 2013 to 2025," Report Prepared for the Association of American Medical Colleges, March 2015, https://www.aamc.org/download/426242/data/ihsreportdownload.pdf?cm_mmc= AAMC-_-ScientificAffairs-_-PDF-_-ihsreport.

States should also modernize physician licensing. Nonreciprocal licensing by states unnecessarily limits patient care, especially as telemedicine proliferates. It is also time to relax tight limits to physician supply that have stagnated medical school graduation numbers for almost forty years and bring to light the strictly controlled residency training practices in place for decades. And increasing physician supply is not only necessary for primary care. Almost two-thirds of the doctor shortage of 124,000 projected for the year 2025 will be in specialist areas, not in primary care[8] (Figure 7.1). Residency training programs still find it extraordinarily difficult to increase the number of their trainees, even when paying fully for the additional residency positions. Medical socie-ties that set restrictive quotas harm consumers by artificially limiting the supply of doctors and consequently restricting com-petition among doctors. These anticonsumer practices need to be open to public scrutiny and abolished.

In reality, virtually all patients with serious diseases today are cared for by specialists. For seniors, visits to specialists have increased from 37 percent of visits two decades ago to 55 percent today.[9] And that is appropriate, because specialists are the doctors who have the necessary training and expertise to use the complex diagnostics, new procedures, and novel drugs of modern medicine. To increase the supply of doctors who are trained to use advanced technology and to ensure clinical innovation, we must keep attract-ing top students into medicine. Specific estimates vary, but while the direct payments for malpractice amount to less than 1 percent of health spending, if one includes the $45 billion in costs of defen-sive medicine, the total tallies 2.4 percent of health care spend-ing, or more than $55 billion per year.[10] Therefore, we need to rein in malpractice lawsuits that waste money and discourage pursuit of careers in top specialties and encourage streamlined train-ing when possible. Then, let us add common sense—it would be destructive to artificially determine salaries by government price fixing for those who have the most valuable and unique expertise. Price transparency and more consumer empowerment, prompting competition among providers, more effectively sort out these issues.

Perhaps the most insidious consequence of the ACA is the threat to innovation in drugs, devices, and medical technology—the tools that streamline diagnosis, ensure safer treatment, and save lives. The importance of continuing the stream of new medi-cal technology and highly specialized, targeted treatments can-not be overstated, and, we should note, the overwhelming majority of the world's health care innovations occur in the United States (Figures 7.2 and 7.3; Table 7.1). These innovations include ground-breaking drug treatments, surgical procedures, medical devices,

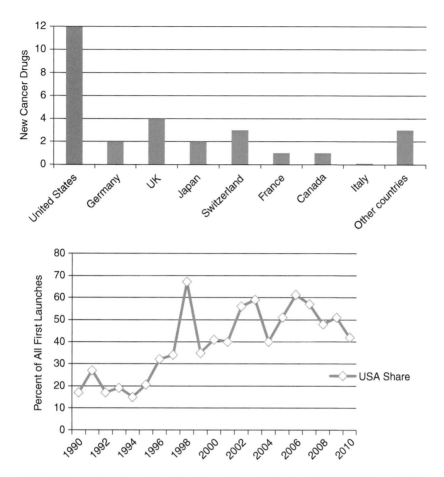

FIGURE 7.2. (*top*) First Launches of New Cancer Drugs by Country, 1995–2005; (*bottom*) US Share of First Launches of New Active Substances, World Market by Year, 1990–2010.
The United States has been the dominant initiator of new drug launches, including new cancer drugs, originating about half of the entire world's new active substances for almost two decades.
Sources: (top): B. Jonsson and N. Wilking, "Market Uptake of New Oncology Drugs," *Annals of Oncology* 18, suppl 3 (2007): iii2–iii7, doi:10.1093/annonc/mdm099; (*bottom*): US Food and Drug Administration, "FY 2011 Innovative Drug Approvals," November 2011, http://www.fda.gov /downloads/AboutFDA/ReportsManualsForms/Reports/UCM278358.pdf.

patents, diagnostics, and much more. A recent *R&D Magazine* survey of research and development (R&D) leaders from sixty-three countries ranked the United States No. 1 in the world for health care innovation.

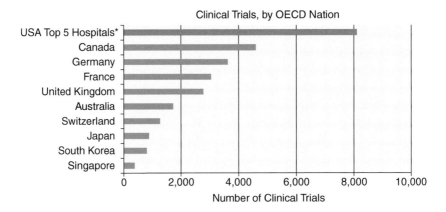

FIGURE 7.3. Clinical Trials, by OECD Nation.
The top five US hospitals conduct more clinical trials than any OECD nation.
Note: *Top five US hospitals as ranked by *US News and World Report,* 2007.
Source: McKinsey Global Institute, "Accounting for the Cost of US Health Care: A New Look at Why Americans Spend More," December 2008, http://www.mckinsey.com/insights/health _systems_and_services/accounting_for_the_cost_of_us_health_care.

But that environment is changing. Growth of total US R&D expenditures from 2012 to 2014 averaged only 2.1 percent, down from an average of 6 percent over the previous fifteen years.[11] Although the slowdown is partly attributable to the weak economy since the 2008 financial crisis, it has been exacerbated by Obamacare's new taxes and regulations. According to CBO estimates, the law will impose more than $500 billion in new taxes over its first decade to help pay for its insurance subsidies and Medicaid expansion. These taxes include significant ones on key health care industries, including manufacturers of medical devices and drugs and their investors. Because of the Obamacare tax burden, small and large US health care technology companies are moving R&D centers and jobs overseas. Already a long list of such companies—including Boston Scientific, Stryker, and Cook Medical—have announced job cuts and new centers overseas for R&D, manufacturing, and clinical trials.

Bureaucracy at the FDA is also hindering medical technology and drug development. Developing new drugs now takes about fourteen years and costs more than $2.5 billion.[12] According to a

TABLE 7.1 Major Medical Innovations and Country of Origin

Rank	Technology	Description	Country of Origin
1	Magnetic resonance imaging	Noninvasive diagnostic imaging	USA, UK
	Computed tomography		USA, UK
2	Angiotensin-converting enzyme inhibitors	Drugs for hypertension and heart failure	USA
3	Balloon angioplasty	Minimally invasive surgery to unblock arteries	Switzerland
4	Statins	Cholesterol-reducing drugs	USA, Japan
5	Mammography	Breast cancer detection	Indeterminate
6	Coronary artery bypass graft surgery	Surgery for heart failure	USA
7	Proton pump inhibitors	Antiulcer drugs	Sweden, USA
8	Selective serotonin reuptake inhibitors	Antidepressant drugs	USA
9	Cataract extraction and lens implant	Eye surgery	USA
10	Hip replacement	Mechanical prostheses	UK
	Knee replacement		Japan, UK, USA

Source: Based on V. Fuchs and H. Sox, "Physicians' Views of the Relative Importance of 30 Medical Innovations," Health Affairs 20 (2001): 30–42.

2010 survey of more than two hundred medical technology companies, delays for approvals of new devices are now far longer than in Europe.[13] In the European Union—not exactly known for minimizing red tape—it takes seven months on average to gain approval for low- to moderate-risk devices. In the United States, FDA approval time averages thirty-one months. PricewaterhouseCooper's 2011 Innovation Scorecard for medical technology found a worsening in the United States over the past five years. The report stated that "although the United States will hold its lead, the country will continue to lose ground during the next decade."[14] Meanwhile, emerging nations such as India and China have significantly improved their own environments for innovation and entrepreneurs.

What can be done to reverse these damaging trends? First, strip back the heavy tax burdens on industries and investors that inhibit innovation, starting with repealing the ACA's $24 billion medical device excise tax and the $30 billion tax on brand-name drugs. Repeal the Obamacare investment tax to restore tax incentives for essential funding of early stage medical technology and life science companies. And simplify processes for new device and drug approvals so that the FDA becomes a favorable rather than an obstructionist environment for life-saving and cost-saving discoveries, as well as a facilitator for the availability of lower-cost generics.

Finally, intelligent immigration reforms are needed to encourage educated, highly skilled entrepreneurs to stay in the United States. Many of the best and brightest who come to the United States to study science, technology, engineering, and math—subjects crucial to health care innovation—are now choosing to return to their home countries after they finish their studies. In contrast to a decade ago, when from 66 percent to more than 90 percent of foreign students studying in the United States remained here after they completed their studies, only 6 percent of Indian, 10 percent of Chinese, and 15 percent of European students expect to make America their permanent home today.[15] Although some of this shift is undoubtedly the result of improving opportunities in those students' home countries and other incentives for them to return home, many graduates want to remain in the United States but are unable to do so. Lawmakers should take a fresh look at easing counterproductive immigration restrictions. New skills-based visa programs should be instituted that specifically target highly educated individuals, particularly students completing American university graduate-degree programs in the areas of science, technology, engineering, and math.

Conclusion

Even if one recognizes the unsurpassed excellence of medical care that has been widely available in the United States, reforms are urgent, particularly in light of the deleterious impacts of Obamacare. Costs are high and escalating; government expenditures will soon overwhelm the entire federal budget in the absence of change. This situation causes great concern about the sustainability of access to medical care and its excellence for Americans in the long term. Reforms to the system are essential—the debate is about what specific reforms are appropriate to fix the inadequacies and reduce the cost without jeopardizing its excellence and without stifling innovation.

Paradoxically, as Obamacare is doubling down on government authority over health care, the solution in those countries with the longest experience of nationalized health care, from Britain to Denmark to Sweden, is increasingly to shift patients toward private health care to remedy their failed systems.[1] Likewise, Europeans with means or power are increasingly circumventing their centralized health systems. Private insurance in the European Union has grown by more than 50 percent in the past decade.[2] In reaction to their unconscionable waits for care,[3] about 11 percent of Britons hold private health insurance, including almost two-thirds who earn more than $78,700—even though they are already paying taxes to the tune of £114 billion ($175 billion) for their "free" National Health Service insurance[4] and despite the government's sharp rise in an insurance premium tax to thwart private insurance.[5] In Sweden, despite the fact that an average family already pays nearly $20,000 annually in taxes toward health care, almost

600,000 Swedes now use private insurance, a number that has increased by 67 percent over the last five years.[6] Unless Obamacare is drastically altered, America's health care will also become even more divided. If sustained, it will be driven toward two parallel systems with even more inequality; as in the United Kingdom and elsewhere, only the lower and middle classes in America will suffer the full harm of Obamacare.

As outlined herein, specific reforms that would improve the availability for all Americans to high-quality care and would reduce costs without damaging the excellence of America's medical care are within reach. Using specific incentives and detailed proposals, the plan I suggest enhances the availability and affordability of twenty-first-century medical care and ensures continued health care innovation. These reforms promise to be disruptive and drive important efficiencies into health care. Once the reforms are fully implemented, the quality of health care will improve, and total national health spending will substantially decrease, generating significant savings and increased economic activity into other areas of the US economy. Modernizing US health care should center on expanding high-deductible insurance coverage and health savings accounts. These fundamental reforms expand the purchasing power of consumers, the necessary basis for enhancing market competition that will ultimately lead to better value and more consumer choices. And voters overwhelmingly support such reforms. In answer to the question, "What would do more to reduce health care costs—more free market competition between insurance companies or more government regulation?," 62 percent of voters chose more free market competition, and only 26 percent chose more regulation.[7] A vast majority of Americans—a full 73 percent—say they have a right to choose between health insurance plans that cost more and cover just about all medical procedures versus other plans that cost less while covering only major medical procedures (only 12 percent are opposed).[8] An even greater majority, 85 percent to only 7 percent, say individuals should have the right to choose between health plans that have higher deduct-ibles and lower premiums versus plans with lower deductibles and higher premiums. It is the responsibility of government leaders to work to create health reforms that reflect these important princi-ples held by the American people.

Key Questions and Answers on the Atlas Plan

The State of US Health Care

If the US health care system was so good before Obamacare, then why does US life expectancy lag behind so many other countries?

- Life expectancy figures are poor indicators of health system quality (see Scott W. Atlas, "The Limited Value of Life Expectancy Comparisons in Ranking Health Systems," in *In Excellent Health: Setting the Record Straight on America's Health Care*, Hoover Press, 2011). Many factors significantly impact overall life expectancy; many have little or nothing to do with quality of health care. For example, the United States ranked near the bottom of the life expectancy tables compiled by the OECD, an international organization whose members include the world's economically developed nations. Then, in 2007, Ohsfeldt and Schneider standardized countries for all immediate deaths from homicide, suicide, and high-speed motor vehicle accidents (situations where health care is irrelevant). The United States moved to the top of the ranking! Personal lifestyle choices involving nutrition, exercise, obesity, cigarette smoking, and safe sexual practices impact life expectancy. The United States has a greater commitment to caring for vulnerable newborns and senior citizens. Individual decisions to follow doctor recommendations about treatments, follow-up, and prescribed medications all influence life expectancy.
- Countries differ greatly in their population heterogeneity, which strongly influences mortality rates due to genetic susceptibility to disease, socioeconomic variations, differences in education,

and other factors separate from the quality of medical care. Differences in technology, disposable income, violence, urbanization, marriage rates, and economic inequality also change life expectancy. Some of these factors bias the statistic against US life expectancy because the United States has the world's largest historical burden of smoking and rising obesity, the two major lifestyle risk factors for premature death, independent of health care quality. The OECD estimates that the lifespan of an obese person is up to eight to ten years shorter than that of a normal-weight person, matching the loss of longevity seen in cigarette smokers.

If the US health care system was so good before Obamacare, then why is the US infant mortality rate worse than that of so many other countries?

■ The infant mortality rate is a complex and multifactorial end point that oversimplifies multiple inputs, many of which have no tie to health care at all. It is plagued by widely varying definitions of key terms, registration biases, and a large number of risk factors that distort the final statistic, all of which render the figure invalid as a comparison measure of health care. And the United States is different from other countries in important ways regarding infant mortality, including the following: (1) the United States adheres strictly to World Health Organization's definition of "live births" and records all births, whereas most other countries do not count high-risk newborns who die early; (2) medical standards differ among countries; for example, the United States uniquely prioritizes a "full-court press" to resuscitate and save even the most premature infants with the least likelihood of survival; and (3) the United States has the highest frequency of preterm births, the dominant risk factor for neonatal mortality (these factors and others are reviewed in detail in Scott W. Atlas, "Infant Mortality as an Indicator of Health and

Health Care," *In Excellent Health: Setting the Record Straight on America's Health Care*, Hoover Press, 2011).

Expanding Affordable Private Insurance

Did Obamacare improve anything about private insurance? If so, does this plan keep those features?

- Yes—Obamacare eliminated lifetime caps on total benefits and prevented insurers from dropping already insured people if they became diagnosed with a disease. Obamacare also put in place annual out-of-pocket maximums. These features would be maintained in this plan.

Is there a mandate in the Atlas plan forcing individuals to purchase health insurance?

- No—no one is forced to buy health insurance or penalized for not buying it. Despite the failure of the Roberts Supreme Court to stop such a mandate, it is not the role of the US government to force Americans to purchase a good or service they do not want. That is both anticompetitive and anticonsumer. And there is another reason—mandates are typically not very effective and quite complicated to enforce. The decades of experience in the United States with mandates for automobile insurance and even income taxes show that mandates have a 14 percent to 18 percent noncompliance rate—a percentage strikingly similar to the percentage cited as uninsured without any mandate. You may have also noticed all of the unanswered questions and concerns about enforcement of the Obamacare mandate and, equally important, the massive number of waivers being granted since its implementation for temporary political gain.
- My plan takes a different approach—it brings incentives to the system to generate insurance products that are more in line with

what consumers want and gives consumers incentives to buy those products. This way, consumers will purchase the coverage (and health care) that they think is a good value. After all, the money belongs to individuals and their families, not to the government.

But what about the "free riders" who don't buy insurance? Aren't those of us who buy insurance paying a lot more for our premiums because of them?

■ No—this is one of the great myths behind the idea of forcing everyone to buy insurance. We all care about "fairness," but facts are important. In reality, as Hadley showed in 2008, "private insurance premiums are at most 1.7 percent higher because of the shifting of costs of the uninsured"; if a more realistic estimate of cost shifting is used, premiums are less than 1 percent higher due to the shift from people without insurance. This impact is very minimal.

Under the Atlas plan, would I be refused care at the emergency room if I have no health insurance?

■ No—my plan does not change the laws protecting uninsured patients. Since the 1986 Emergency Medical Treatment and Active Labor Act, hospitals cannot turn away any individual seeking medical care—regardless of insurance status or ability to pay. Even decades before this law, safeguards for uninsured patients already existed. According to Hadley in 2008, $86 billion per year of medical care is administered to the uninsured. Roughly $43 billion is paid by federal, state, and local governments; another $30 billion or so is paid out of pocket. America's doctors contribute another $8 billion per year in free charity care. And contrary to popular belief, free care is given not only through the emergency room in emergency circumstances; a full 86 percent of free care is given through offices and clinics.

Won't the uninsured people clog up emergency rooms and cause a great financial burden on the rest of us who have insurance?

■ No—first, the recent Oregon study showed that when uninsured people become insured, they use the emergency room more frequently, not less. This finding contradicts the theory that uninsured people overutilize emergency rooms and, with that, shift costs to the insured. Second, the estimated cost shift from the uninsured to insurance premiums paid by the insured is less than 1 percent, that is, a very small amount. This situation will not disappear under my proposal, but it will diminish because (1) more of the poor will have incentives to enroll in coverage (to protect their new assets in HSAs), and (2) the cost of care and insurance will be lower.

If everyone used high-deductible insurance, wouldn't that eliminate coverage for preventive care and screening and require out-of-pocket payment?

■ No—nearly all high-deductible insurance already covered those visits and procedures, that is, they are not subject to deductibles. My plan does not change this. The real problem is that most enrollees are not aware of this.

What about office visits to doctors? Are they covered in this plan?

■ Yes—every limited-mandate plan will include three routine office visits per year that are not subject to any deductible. This is unchanged from the catastrophic insurance coverage under Obamacare.

Would the new insurance plans require copays?

■ The new plans would be designed by the insurers, not by my plan or the government, so a variety of arrangements is likely.

Consumers would decide what coverage suits their needs, just like consumers decide what food to buy, what sort of clothing and shelter they desire, and what level of safety features they value in a car. Individuals would purchase coverage with the level of copayments that they personally value. As with all other goods and services in a free market, the private sector responds to consumer demands by designing products that will sell, and explaining the benefits of those products, to meet the demands of the empowered buyers.

Limited-mandate catastrophic coverage would not cover some aspects of medical care that many people want covered by insurance. How would people pay for that type of care under the Atlas plan?

■ People who want coverage for treatments such as chiropractic care, or acupuncture, or even marriage therapy and massage, that is, any benefits not included in LMCC, are still free to purchase more comprehensive coverage. Just as with other sorts of products, if consumers want to purchase products with added features, the free market is always interested in selling those added features. Plans covering all those benefits will remain available, just like today, but the premiums for those expensive policies will not be tax deductible. Alternatively, people who value that type of service could pay out of pocket from their HSA balances when that service is desired.

Aren't you forcing people to buy a specific type of insurance?

■ No—my plan does not force anyone to buy any insurance—there is no mandate or penalty coercing anyone to buy any form of health coverage. My plan increases choices for consumers instead of forcing people to buy insurance coverage for services that many people do not want and would never use. Instead of mandates, my proposal provides financial incentives to buy low-cost catastrophic coverage. The catastrophic coverage that this reform package encourages is insurance that has already proved to be a good value because consumers have increasingly moved to purchase this type of insurance when it has been available. In addition, my plan will generate more options for individuals. This plan will reduce the cost of medical care, consequently lowering the cost of insurance. Insurers will respond to the new environment where there are fewer restrictions on insurance plans and where consumers are free to look for insurance tailored to their personal goals for coverage.

Under the Atlas plan, could I be dropped from my insurance if I get a serious disease?

- Americans who stay in continuous insurance coverage should not be penalized for developing costly diseases. In my plan, you cannot be dropped from coverage if you acquire or harbor a disease once insured; this feature serves as another incentive to become insured and then maintain insured status.

But could I buy insurance in the Atlas plan if I already have a disease, and I did not have insurance beforehand?

- Yes—but it would probably cost you significantly more money than if you had bought it beforehand. You are referring to the rules put in place by Obamacare. Obamacare required "guaranteed issue" of insurance. Obamacare prohibited insurers in the individual market from denying coverage, increasing premiums, or restricting benefits because of any preexisting condition. Those rules are actually bad for consumers. First, the rules provided an incentive to those who simply avoided paying for insurance until they acquired a serious disease. This is unfair to everyone else, especially those who took the personal responsibility and bought insurance while they were healthy in anticipation of possibly needing insurance to protect against the financial risk of becoming ill. Second, we knew from states' experience with "guaranteed issue" that two things would happen: coverage would become less available because carriers would leave the market, and premiums would increase for everyone else. States with those regulations are typically those with the least affordable health insurance (The Most Affordable Cities for Children's & Family Health Insurance, 2006). The young and healthy—typically those who earn the least and are most likely to be uninsured—are forced to subsidize the rates of older and often wealthier individuals, which also interferes with risk pools. Under Obamacare, new "guaranteed issue" rules increased insurance premiums by about 20–45 percent, according to Milliman's report of 2013. My plan is fairer for everyone and better for consumers. It rewards people for being responsible and maintaining insurance so that they cannot be dropped once they become ill.

- In my plan, states will form high-risk pools using new models to help those with diseases buy more affordable insurance. For instance, as a condition for selling insurance in a given state market, private health insurance companies would establish a risk-pooling cooperative into which they would pay premiums to protect against the risk of very high health claims. Premiums would be related to the actuarial value of the risk characteristics of their enrollee populations. Perhaps even more important, my plan would lower the cost of insurance for everyone, so more people would be able to afford health insurance before they became ill in the first place.

Under the Atlas plan, will I lose my Obamacare subsidy to purchase private insurance on Obamacare exchanges?

- Yes—but the $850 billion of Obamacare subsidies given to help pay for private insurance under the ACA is necessary because the law itself caused prices of private insurance to skyrocket. My plan is more sensible—I remove many of the factors (for example, excessive mandates) that caused the cost of coverage to become so expensive. Under my plan, insurance coverage will become far less expensive, so people will be able to afford the insurance and actually choose to pay for it because it represents a good value. In addition, take-home wages will increase from the tax reforms in my plan, so Americans will have more money for themselves to spend how they choose.

Won't I lose my employer-provided health benefit if the income exclusion is capped that low?

■ No—under my plan, the maximum allowable health benefit provided by employers will be set to match the maximum allowed for an HSA under my plan. That benefit is fully deductible for the employer and the employee under my plan. In addition, economists generally agree that the employer-employee market trades benefits for wages, which, in the long run, implies that employers would be forced by competition to raise wages commensurate with reduced benefits. Employees would receive higher take-home pay.

Won't the Atlas plan, with its removal of certain tax subsidies and other changes, result in millions of people becoming uninsured?

■ No—the reforms in this plan will markedly increase the consumer's purchasing power for medical care, and this increase will more than compensate for the loss of tax subsidies for purchasing health care or insurance. The prices of health care will decrease as competition ensues and as the counterproductive, perverse incentives in our current system are removed. In my plan, the idea is to generate insurance options that people value and therefore decide to purchase, rather than force people under threat of penalty to buy insurance products that they would not choose to spend their money on.

What about prescription drugs, especially for people with chronic diseases? How will they pay for their medications?

■ All limited-mandate plans will also include coverage for prescription drugs. And people will still have the same options to buy coverage that includes lower deductibles or even exempts drugs from being subject to deductibles. My plan will result in more choices of insurance coverage, not less. That is what experience shows in all other goods or services in a free market—the private sector ultimately supplies products that consumers want to buy; consumers have the control of the money in my plan. Even today, some states already include plans with separate (lower) deductibles for prescription drugs; my plan will probably result in even more of these tailored deductibles.

Why doesn't this plan place price caps on prescription drugs, so patients can afford them?

■ Price caps ultimately do not work to provide the desired products at lower prices. In fact, price caps restrict the availability of the product—this is "Econ 101." In this case, it would do great harm to patients to impose such caps because the number of drugs would become less available, and, even if available, they would be in scarce supply. My reforms would reduce the costs of drugs by virtue of the following: unleashing the power of consumers with control of payments; ridding our system of the regulatory excesses that generate the massive costs and time involved in new drug discovery; streamlining the overly long approval process for lower-cost generic drugs; eliminating the punitive taxes on the pharmaceutical industry that are passed on to consumers; and reversing the Obamacare elements that have contributed to the ongoing consolidation that will further harm consumers. The biggest danger for Americans, particularly senior citizens, who commonly depend on prescription drugs, is increasing insurer consolidation and even more control by the government over decisions on insurance reimbursement. As proved by history and by those countries with government-centralized health care, more government domination over health care results in less access to the life-saving drugs that government bureaucrats judge to be costly or "unnecessary." For example, we see this in such systems as the National Health Service in England and in Canada, with their scandalous waiting lists, limitations on innovative drugs and tests, and worse outcomes than here in the United States.

Why pick on obesity?

■ Obesity is the most serious public health problem in the United States in terms of both its costs and its harmful impact on health. Just like cigarette smoking, obesity is a high-risk voluntary lifestyle for most individuals and a major driver of health expense with well-known health hazards. As is the case for virtually every other form of insurance, rates for health insurance that reflect the higher risk of disease and more frequent use of medical care as a consequence of voluntary behavior are totally appropriate. Risky driving is a key factor in determining automobile insurance rates. Although difficult to do, the way to eliminate most cases is well known and in the hands of individuals. My plan does not discriminate against people who are obese; in fact, it extends more help to those who need it, with more wellness programs, including nutritional counseling and exercise training.

Establishing and Expanding Universal Health Savings Accounts

The Atlas plan eliminates the requirement for a government-defined deductible in order to open an HSA. Is any health insurance required to fund the HSA? If so, what type?

- Yes—to be eligible to contribute to an HSA in any given year, you must also have insurance that covers catastrophic care. My plan does not specify the level of deductible, though—the only contingency is that catastrophic care is covered.

But isn't the purpose of the HSA to cover the high deductible so that health expenses that are smaller than the deductible are paid by the HSA?

- That's partly true. Money in an HSA could also be used for copays, for example, but not for insurance premiums. The new limits on contributions to HSAs would roughly equal the maximum allowed for annual out-of-pocket spending, including deductibles and copays (and those maximums would increase as indexed to the consumer price index). But it might also be valuable to have money in the HSA to pay for medical services that may not be covered by the new insurance plan. Remember, many people will probably buy a limited-mandate plan because it would be cheaper. At some point, an enrollee might want to use an uncovered medical service; that could be paid out of the HSA. And, finally, take-home wages will be higher because employers will shift much of the previous payments for tax-preferred benefits to direct wages because of the tax reforms under this plan.

How specifically are the new HSAs liberalized for more uses?

- First, expenditures from new HSAs would be permitted not only for the account holder but also for spouses, children, parents, and siblings—regardless of the tax dependency of those family members on the named account holder. Current law permits expenses only for the account holder, spouse, and tax-dependent children. Second, expenditures for proven over-the-counter medications will be permitted under new HSAs. Current law limits HSA expenditures to prescription drugs and insulin.

Why wouldn't people just withdraw money from HSAs for other uses?

- It is true that money could be withdrawn from HSAs for noneligible uses. The financial penalty for withdrawals of funds from HSAs will be significant, however—it will be raised to 50 percent from the current 20 percent. More important, most insurance under my plan will likely have a high deductible, so it will be important for everyone to save money in the HSA for health care expenditures.

Do you get to keep the HSA as a tax-sheltered account even if you drop the insurance plan after you have established and funded the HSA?

- Yes—this is the law today, and this plan does not change it.

Would seniors be allowed to withdraw from their HSAs for other reasons outside of health care without penalty?

- Once age seventy, seniors would be allowed to withdraw from their HSAs without the full 50 percent penalty. Nevertheless, the HSA is not intended to be a retirement account for expenditures other than health care. In new Medicare HSAs, a 20 percent penalty would be in place for non-health-care withdrawals, starting once the owner of the HSA became seventy years old. And these accounts will now be able to be passed on to living family members without penalty.

People can't really shop for medical care—it's too complicated, isn't it?

- No, it is not too complicated for most individuals—as long as the information necessary to make informed decisions is visible, then shopping for nonemergency medical care would be simple.

We know that Americans find it straightforward to shop for computers and other far more complicated items. Under my plan, price transparency and competition create even more visible information for consumers. And remember, most medical care episodes are not an "emergency" where life-and-death decisions must be made quickly.

If everyone had a new HSA at birth, who would keep track of those accounts?

■ The federal government would be the repository of the information. This is already true—the federal government regulates and keeps track of all HSAs today.

Instilling Appropriate Incentives through Rational Tax Reforms

Why not allow income tax exclusions or deductions for all insurance, including low-deductible insurance, if the premiums are low (that is, why not just cap the level of the deduction)?

■ The purpose of my tax reform is not solely to cap the amount of the deduction (or income exclusion). It would be counterproductive to allow a tax preference for insurance that covers care by hiding the costs of that care—that is a fundamental cause of rising costs. I want to put the consideration of value and price back into the consumer's purchasing decisions, just as value and price are considered in every other good and service. My plan reforms health insurance back to the way it was intended to function, that is, to cover only *significant* and unexpected costs. That way, individuals would have the power—because they pay directly (up to the deductible), they shop for value, and market forces will reduce costs of care down to what consumers determine would be a good value for their money.

What level of deductible does the Atlas plan use to define an insurance plan as "high deductible"?

- My definition of "high deductible" is based on 75 percent of the maximum allowable HSA contribution. For example, to qualify as a high-deductible plan for 2016, during which the allowable HSA contribution will be $6,850, the definition of high deductible equals $5,137.50. This linkage ensures that the HSA contribution maximum will always potentially be higher than covering just the deductible.

Why is the specific amount of $6,850 chosen for the maximum tax exclusion?

- Although like all such thresholds, the selection of such a number is somewhat arbitrary, this number was chosen for a few reasons: (1) it matches the currently allowed annual out-of-pocket expenses under the ACA; (2) it matches the proposed maximum for deductible HSA annual contribution; and (3) it approximates the average annual employer-based health benefit.

Why not allow a tax deduction for all health care spending instead of limiting the tax preference to HSAs and high-deductible insurance premiums?

- Tax deductions for all health care spending give an incentive to spend more money on health care; in other words, there is an opportunity cost if you spend money on something other than health care because the money is worth more when spent on health care. That preference generates more and more spending on health care rather than on other desired goods and services. My plan eliminates that misincentive. Instead, the incentive is to put money into an HSA and then seek value when it is spent on necessary care; the opportunity cost is when it is spent because it could be saved and then grow by investment (or bequeathed to the account owner's survivors).

Won't the tax preference for basic catastrophic coverage cause higher prices for that coverage because of subsequent increased demand?

- Generally, high demand for goods does lead to price increases. However, increasing demand for the insurance itself is not a significant driver of the cost of insurance premiums. Health insurance premiums rise mainly in response to increases in the cost of providing health care services, not demand for the insurance itself. Prior and anticipated payouts for medical services are by far the single largest component of health insurance premiums. When the cost of health care services increases, insurance premiums rise. Other factors do have some impact on private insurance premiums, including government regulations, in particular mandated coverage; characteristics of the insured individual (for example, age and certain behaviors); and cost shifting caused by underpayment by public insurance. We need to recognize that the main reason for the lower premiums of catastrophic coverage with high deductibles and fewer mandates lies in the very structure of limited-mandate coverage. Premiums of high-deductible catastrophic coverage are lower than premiums of so-called comprehensive coverage because of the anticipated lower costs of covering the medical care under the plan.

Won't the new tax reforms hurt the middle class?

- No—my tax reforms specifically help the middle class and target more affluent individuals. The current tax preference is unfair—it gives a high-value tax deduction for high spending on health insurance that covers everything without limits. This feature overwhelmingly benefits the upper-income earners, that is, the people who enjoy the biggest value from the present tax deduction. The existing tax preference gives a disproportionate benefit to the wealthy because of their higher marginal tax bracket. My plan simplifies the tax reform and removes the special benefit that high-income earners accrue from the current tax exclusion. Ultimately, the cost of insurance premiums and medical care will be reduced by this plan more than the tax benefit for health spending that has distorted the market for health care.

■ As of 2018, the ACA institutes a new "Cadillac tax"—a 40 percent tax on expensive health insurance plans. But the logic for that tax approaches absurdity. Obamacare assesses a new tax on health insurance that exceeds a certain price. Obamacare by its regulations simultaneously caused the prices of health insurance to rise. Therefore, the government ends up imposing a tax on insurance whose price became high, and consequently subject to the tax, directly because of the government's own policy to begin with. In addition, the Cadillac tax will count HSA contributions (from employers and individuals) toward the threshold for invoking the tax penalty, thereby penalizing consumers for trying to keep health care costs low.

■ My tax plan is simpler and also fairer to everyone because it levels the playing field. Under my plan, small business employees, part-time workers, and self-employed people will all have the same deduction as those working for large employers. My plan also gives a tax deduction for significantly expanded HSA contributions, which will increase everyone's savings for out-of-pocket medical costs. Moreover, this plan will help the middle class with more affordable insurance coverage and more control of costs because they have new purchasing power.

Won't the new tax reforms hurt employees by reducing benefits because employers will lose some of their deductions for health benefits?

■ No—the truth is that to a large extent employees pay for their benefits by receiving lower wages than they would have otherwise been paid. Employment benefits, including health care benefits, replace wages. If I limit the tax deduction for health benefits paid by employers, then employers would likely pay less of those benefits at first. But over time, employees will instead receive higher wages and more take-home pay as employers are forced to compete with higher wages to attract labor.

Won't reducing the allowable income exclusion from taxation constitute a new tax increase and therefore reduce wages?

■ No—this six-point health reform plan will reduce the medical care costs by more than the lost value of the old tax exclusion for health benefits to consumers. The proposed tax reform herein is a cut in a tax expenditure program (see *Fiscal Year 2016 Analytical Perspectives of the US Government of the Federal Budget*, p. 255). In addition, the reforms in this plan will increase take-home wages as employer behavior changes in response to the health reform plan.

Modernizing Medicare for the Twenty-First Century

Isn't this plan going to destroy Medicare?

■ No—quite the opposite. My plan will introduce competition among insurance companies, so cheaper insurance options will become available for consumers. This plan will expand choices for beneficiaries, so beneficiaries can decide whether they want more comprehensive coverage or lower-cost insurance coverage. It also helps seniors allocate more savings to cover out-of-pocket expenses through new eligibility for expanded HSAs, and it allows seniors more flexibility on paying for those health-related items from their HSAs. This plan will significantly reduce the cost of Medicare so that it will be available for generations to come. And this long-term viability is crucial because Medicare will be even more important in the future, as more people live longer and medical advances continue. In the long run, traditional Medicare will be moved to private health insurance to improve benefits, reduce costs, and eliminate the increasing problem of seniors of finding doctors and hospitals who accept Medicare. For those over age thirty-five today, though, traditional Medicare will still be an option when they become Medicare eligible.

How is this Medicare reform different from previous reform proposals?

■ This plan shares some key principles of reform with prior proposals, most notably the fundamental idea of defined benefits for premium support and competition among insurers for enrollees. Still, this plan differs from previous proposals in a number of important ways, including the following:

- The benchmark used to calculate Medicare's payment for premiums would be determined by an average of the three lowest-priced private plans submitted; included in those would be a limited-mandate plan.
- New Medicare would contain a major expansion and liberalization of HSAs, including new eligibility for universal HSA ownership and continuing contributions for all beneficiaries; significant expansion of HSA limits; broader HSA uses; new rules allowing transfers from retirement accounts; and new permission to pass on HSA balances to surviving family members.
- While everyone over age thirty-five today will still have the option of traditional Medicare, eventually traditional Medicare coverage would be phased out entirely so that ultimately all Medicare beneficiaries would have the advantages of private insurance, with better access to doctors, hospitals, drug treatments, and advanced medical technology.
- Instead of sharing rebates with the government after choosing cheaper insurance (as happens today with Medicare

Advantage), new Medicare beneficiaries would receive 100 percent of the rebates, in cash returns to their HSAs, if they selected insurance with lower premiums than the benchmark.

- The plan would eliminate the current anticonsumer conflict of interest of the federal government that allows government restrictions on access to medical care. Today, with its role as the insurer via traditional Medicare, the government has the power to restrict access to care and artificially set prices of medical services. This ability has already caused a reduction in doctor acceptance of Medicare, and trends show further reductions. Under my plan, traditional Medicare is eliminated, so the government will support beneficiaries with money to buy insurance instead of dictating benefits and prices as an insurer. In the new Medicare, the government will stay out of the way of impeding consumer choice and access to care. With the new plan, the Medicare patient will have the power to choose from the same wide array and state-of-the-art excellence of medical care as everyone else.

How will the Atlas reforms of Medicare deal with risk pools and adverse selection, where some insurers will mainly enroll low-risk, healthier seniors and create far more expensive insurance for those with chronic diseases?

- A risk pool is the basic foundation of health insurance so that enrollees with lower health care costs offset enrollees with higher health care costs in a large group of enrollees in a given health plan. It is used to spread risk among groups of people enrolled in health plans to allow insurers to manage their ability to pay claims and provide benefits. Insurance markets could be destabilized by a phenomenon called "adverse selection," where sicker individuals enroll in certain plans in a disproportionate number. This causes higher premiums, which in turn cause younger, healthier people to leave the plan, creating a cycle ultimately leading to collapse. Risk pooling is necessary to prevent such spirals. One possible risk pool mechanism would be a risk-adjustment program similar to those proposed by both the Wyden-Ryan plan and the Heritage Foundation's proposal (for more on these plans, see Robert E. Moffit, "Saving the American Dream: Comparing Medicare Reforms Plans" [Heritage Foundation Backgrounder No. 2675, April 4, 2012], http://www .heritage.org/research/reports/2012/04/saving-the-american -dream-comparing-medicare-reform-plans). Participating insurers would be required to establish a national risk pool in order to sell to Medicare beneficiaries. Insurers with higher shares of low-cost enrollees would contribute to a fund that would make payments to insurers with larger shares of high-cost enrollees. Medicare administrators would monitor the enrollment data of participating health plans and require cross subsidies to compensate for plans with a disproportionate enrollment of high-risk beneficiaries. I believe the actual premium changes and calculations of cross subsidies should be performed by the insurers themselves, rather than the government.

How will the coverage of new Medicare insurance plans be determined?

■ The coverage and benefits of the new insurance plans will ultimately be determined by the individuals selecting the plans, that is, the Medicare beneficiaries themselves. Under the new Medicare plan, the beneficiaries will have far more choices at competitive prices. Today, overly bloated requirements of coverage that many beneficiaries do not want are causing excessively high premiums and out-of-pocket costs, including the coverage requirements of traditional Medicare. Because beneficiaries would receive rebates into their HSAs if they chose cheaper insurance, they would now have incentives to consider carefully what coverage they chose. Remember, enrollees still have the choice of buying insurance with more extensive coverage.

Equally important, as a result of the new competition in place, insurance and medical care itself would cost less under the new reforms to the health care system.

Won't seniors be at greater risk if the government is not the insurer? Who will protect seniors?

■ My plan ensures that seniors will be protected the same way they are now—by the existing Center for Drug and Health Plan Choice, a federal oversight agency that resides within the Centers for Medicare and Medicaid Services. This center would have authority to approve insurance plans that meet standards, just like it does today for Medicare Advantage plans and drug benefit plans competing in today's Part D (nonetheless, it would not have authority to standardize benefits of plans or determine rates). Moreover, the state-based regulatory agencies that currently enforce rules for health insurance and consumer protection against fraud and misleading advertising will also remain in place. This reform plan does nothing to expose seniors to more risk or danger.

What about low-income seniors?

■ Just like today, America's safety net for low-income senior citizens would remain in place for the so-called dual eligible. Medicaid assistance would add to their federal Medicare subsidies. The difference is that under the reforms to both Medicaid and Medicare in this proposal, the choices, the access, and the quality of health care for low-income seniors would be strengthened and expanded.

Will I lose my current doctor whom I have seen for years under Medicare? Seniors have complicated medical problems, so it is very important to have continuity of care.

- No—in fact, my plan will reduce the problem of finding doctors that has already begun. Today, more and more doctors are refusing to see Medicare patients. Traditional Medicare pays doctors less than cost. In my plan, more Medicare patients will be allowed to buy private insurance identical to non-Medicare patients, that is, coverage that pays doctors appropriate amounts for care. The plan eliminates the main reason for doctors dropping Medicare. And the same applies to hospitals. Under this plan, the best hospitals and specialists, the doctors whom seniors need most, will no longer drop Medicare acceptance.

How would beneficiary income be used to determine new Medicare benefits under the Atlas plan?

- My plan is similar to current income adjustments in today's Medicare Part B and Part D, but with some differences. Today, adjusted gross incomes over $85,000 for individuals and $170,000 for joint filers result in higher monthly premiums up to a certain point, with no complete phase-out of taxpayer subsidies. Under my plan, the same phase-in of premiums adjustments would occur (subsidies from taxpayers would decrease for those with incomes above these thresholds), but in addition I suggest that the highest-income earners (those with adjusted gross incomes greater than $1,000,000 for individuals) would receive no subsidies at all.

Will there be a cap on annual out-of-pocket expenses in the new Medicare insurance plans?

- Yes—the maximum allowable out-of-pocket annual expenses for seniors will be matched to the maximum allowable contribution to HSAs. For 2016, that cap will equal $6,850 for self-only coverage and $13,700 for self-and-family coverage, including the deductible. Nevertheless, lower out-of-pocket maximums will likely also be available among the many choices of insurance plans open to seniors in the new Medicare program.

Under the Atlas plan for Medicare, would seniors be at risk of losing coverage for preexisting conditions, and would the "oldest old" of Medicare beneficiaries pay far higher rates?

- No—nothing would change from the current status of community rating (where premiums would be based on the pool of enrollees, not the individual) and guaranteed issue (where existing health problems would not prevent the individual from obtaining insurance) in the current Medicare program. All participating insurance plans would retain current Medicare rules.

What would happen to the complicated rules wherein some doctors accept Medicare assignment and others do not?

- Those rules would be abolished. Under this new plan, Medicare beneficiaries would be allowed to purchase medical care with cash, insurance, or any other means of payment agreeable to them and their doctors. And health care providers could accept any means of payment without the current restrictions that interfere with doctor access for Medicare beneficiaries.

How quickly would the age of eligibility for Medicare increase?

- Two months per year—so it would take six years for the eligibility age to have increased by one year, twelve years for it to have increased by two years, and so forth. And it would only affect those currently age fifty or younger. For example, under the current system, people currently age fifty become eligible for Medicare in fifteen years (in the year 2030). Under my plan, the age of eligibility would increase by thirty months after fifteen years from the implementation of the rule change; therefore, individuals now age fifty would become eligible for Medicare at age

67.5. In the year 2045, that is, in thirty years, the age of eligibility would be seventy. Any subsequent changes in eligibility age would be related to the increases in US life expectancy.

Will prescription drugs and cancer screening be covered in the new Medicare plans accepted for competitive bidding?

- Yes—all Medicare insurance plans will include prescription drug coverage, including limited-mandate catastrophic plans. As they do today, plans will likely require copays, although more choices of coverage and benefits will be available to beneficiaries. All plans will cover the most important cancer screening tests for no out-of-pocket charges, regardless of the deductible.

Given that seniors have much larger health care usage and costs than other age groups, aren't HSAs going to be too small to have any practical value?

- No—under my plan, seniors will have a special allowance to transfer funds from any tax-sheltered retirement account into their HSA without any tax penalty and reversible up to the amount of the transfer. This feature will allow at least some seniors who need a backstop and choose to do so to leverage their new purchasing power for medical care. In addition, seniors who choose coverage that costs less than the benchmark average will receive a rebate into their HSA, that is, money to be used for health care expenses. Lastly, children or other family members will be able to use their HSAs to help pay HSA-eligible expenses. And don't forget that health care itself will cost less.

How do HSA rules under the Atlas Medicare plan differ from current HSA rules for Medicare beneficiaries?

- Under today's Medicare, HSAs are restricted in several ways, many of which are highly complicated and indeed arcane.

- Current HSAs and Medicare:

  - To qualify for an HSA, you cannot be enrolled in Medicare.
  - Beginning with the first month you enroll in Medicare Part A and/or Part B, you can no longer contribute any money to an HSA (you may still withdraw money for eligible expenditures).
  - If you apply for or accept Social Security benefits, even if you continue working, you cannot contribute to an HSA (because once you accept Social Security benefits, you will be automatically enrolled into Medicare Parts A and B). Note that you may decline Medicare Part B if you continue to work for a large employer, but you cannot decline Medicare Part A. Also note that you must stop contributing to your existing HSA six months before you apply for Social Security, or you will owe a tax penalty because Medicare Part A is retroactive for six months prior to the Social Security application.
  - If your spouse is the designated beneficiary, the HSA will be treated as the spouse's HSA at your death; if not, the account stops being an HSA, and its balance becomes taxable to the beneficiary or the estate.

- Current "Medicare Advantage MSAs" (tax-exempt "Archer" medical savings accounts set up with a financial institution into which the Medicare program can deposit money for qualified medical expenses):

  - These accounts are uncommon and offered on a state-by-state basis.
  - Eligibility requires Medicare enrollment *and* enrollment into a high-deductible Medicare Advantage health plan that meets Medicare guidelines.
  - Unlike HSAs, which allow deposits from anyone (yourself, your employer, other family members), neither you nor your employer, if any, are allowed to deposit any money into

Medicare MSAs. Only Medicare can deposit money into your MSA.

- The deposits into Medicare MSAs are generally significantly less than the deductible of the accompanying high-deductible plan, typically less than half.
- In general, you cannot have other health insurance that would cover the cost of services during your Medicare MSA plan's yearly deductible.
- Many people are excluded from Medicare MSA eligibility, including those who have health coverage that would cover the Medicare MSA plan deductible (including benefits from an employer or union group health plan); Medicaid enrollees; those who relocate outside the service area of the plan; and others.
- If you withdraw money for nonqualified expenses, the money becomes taxable, and a 50 percent penalty is charged regardless of the age of the beneficiary.
- If you name a beneficiary for your MSA account who is not your spouse, the money in the account after your death is taxable and added to that person's income when he or she files that year's income tax return.

- Under my new Medicare proposal, the following rules would be in place:

  - All Medicare enrollees are eligible for new Medicare HSAs regardless of enrollment into any or all Medicare coverage.
  - No specific deductible is required on an accompanying insurance plan to contribute to a new Medicare HSA. The only requirement for contributing is having catastrophic coverage, regardless of any level of deductible.
  - Instead of the confusing, complex allowance for those over age sixty-five for HSA spending on certain insurance premiums (that is, can reimburse themselves for the money that Social Security withholds to pay Medicare Part B and can

make tax-free HSA withdrawals to pay Medicare Part D and Medicare Advantage premiums but not Medigap premiums), new HSAs will permit tax-free spending for all premiums of all high-deductible plans.

- New Medicare HSA contribution limits are significantly higher than current HSA limits and current Medicare MSA limits, and they match all other non-Medicare HSA limits.
- New Medicare HSA uses are broadened to match all other non-Medicare HSA uses, including, for example, nonprescription medication.
- New Medicare HSA contributions are open to employers, family members, and individuals.
- New Medicare HSA contributions are allowed even for individuals receiving Social Security benefits.
- Once age seventy, seniors would be allowed to withdraw from their HSAs without the full 50 percent penalty. In new Medicare HSAs, a 20 percent penalty would be in place for non-health-care withdrawals once the owner of the HSA became seventy years old.
- On the death of the senior, new Medicare HSA balances are allowed to be bequeathed to the tax-free HSA of surviving spouses or family members.

Isn't the Atlas plan really just "privatization" of Medicare into a voucher plan?

- Regarding privatization—this plan preserves the federal government benefit of health insurance for senior citizens, with both taxpayer money and administrative oversight by the government. Remember, the reality of current Medicare is that about 75 percent of beneficiaries already supplement or fully replace traditional Medicare with private insurance. Only about 9 percent of beneficiaries have Medicare alone, and another 15 percent or so have both Medicaid and Medicare. The private insurance that will be offered in this new Medicare will have numerous advantages for beneficiaries over the current insurance options, as described elsewhere in this book. Remember also that we already know that the best access to care and the best outcomes from care come from private insurance, not government insurance. This has been proved both here in the United States (for example, the Veterans Health Administration system or Medicaid) and around the globe, where patients in government-centralized systems experience unconscionable waits for care and worse outcomes than care obtained via private insurance. Do not forget another fact—the private insurance of current Medicare Advantage plans outscored traditional Medicare on nine of eleven measures of health care quality in a recent direct comparison (see Brennan and Shepard in 2010 and reviewed in the *New England Journal of Medicine* by Guram and Moffit in 2012). The bottom line is that this reform plan removes government from a position of an inherent conflict of interest—being not only the insurer but also the dominant insurer, with direct or indirect control over nearly all prices and access to care. This fundamental change will increase the availability and quality of medical care and reduce its costs for seniors.

■ Regarding vouchers—no, this is not a voucher plan. In a voucher system, a set amount of money (typically indexed in some way to something that changes over time, such as the consumer price index) is sent to the beneficiary. Then, the beneficiary is basically on his or her own to use it in the purchase of private coverage. My proposal involves premium support, whereby Medicare would pay a certain amount (determined by the Medicare benchmark calculation rather than indexed to anything other than the market price for private insurance by way of competing plans submitted for bid) to a Medicare-approved health plan. In this proposal, seniors are not fending for themselves with vouchers.

Under the Atlas plan, if a beneficiary selects coverage with premiums that are lower than the new Medicare benchmark payment, the beneficiary would receive a rebate. Is that the same as the rebate offered today under Medicare Advantage?

- Not exactly—the proposed plan is more advantageous for consumers. Under current Medicare Advantage, if the selected plan is less than the government's benchmark payment, the plan by law returns 75 percent of the savings to the beneficiary by way of more benefits, and the remaining 25 percent goes to the government. In my plan, the entire amount of the savings—100 percent—goes directly to the consumer in cash, as a deposit to the consumer's HSA; the government would receive nothing.

Overhauling Medicaid to Eliminate the Two-Tiered System

How will the poor get started with HSAs to get into the Atlas health care plan?

- All states will be required to open HSAs for all of their Medicaid enrollees. In addition, states must seed fund at least 50 percent of HSAs belonging to new Medicaid enrollees in order to receive any federal money to support their Medicaid programs. Today, about 57 percent of Medicaid funding comes from the federal government, even though Medicaid is a state-run program, so this condition will be a strong incentive. The second requirement for states to receive federal money for Medicaid is that at least 50 percent of beneficiaries must enroll in limited-mandate private coverage. Under this plan, Medicaid agencies would no longer have direct authority over insurance plans because the plans are private. Agency offices would now assist beneficiaries in finding and enrolling in private plans.

Would current holders of traditional Medicaid suddenly lose their insurance?

- No—they would have the new option of switching to new Medicaid (private high-deductible insurance with money going into their own HSA immediately); in this plan, over a period of ten to twenty years, I envision that traditional Medicaid will be gradually phased out for most Medicaid holders by their own choices. Medicaid will then have been fully transformed into a private insurance premium support program.

Why would doctors suddenly accept new Medicaid patients when they do not accept them now?

- In current traditional Medicaid, the payments for medical services are very low, even below cost in many cases. Under the new plan, doctors and hospitals would receive payments from the same private insurance (or HSAs) as from any other non-Medicaid patient; in the new Medicaid, doctors and hospitals would not even know who was a Medicaid patient and who was not.

What new incentives for healthy lifestyles and preventive care would exist under new Medicaid?

- New Medicaid patients would have the same doctors as private patients. Medicaid patients would receive counsel and the offer of the same screening tests and wellness information as all privately insured patients. In addition, new Medicaid enrollees would have new assets to protect as their HSA balances are built up. The existence of these new assets would provide an incentive for long-term protection. Remember, the rationale for insurance is to cover possible loss of assets; this is also one of the main rationales for receiving preventive care and living a healthy lifestyle.

Increasing the Supply of Medical Care and Ensuring Innovation

Is it realistic to propose streamlined training programs for physicians?

- Yes—innovative, shortened training programs already exist. For example, the NYU School of Medicine has begun offering a streamlined three-year medical degree program. The Texas Tech University School of Medicine and others are also offering accelerated programs.

Why would you call for loosening of immigration limits? Don't immigrants take jobs from American citizens and cost taxpayers money through our public schools and our entitlement programs?

- The immigration reforms suggested in this plan specifically target highly educated, entrepreneurial immigrants who would be here legally. These people are extremely important contributors to American innovation and job creation in our society—they come to the United States for education and opportunity, not for entitlements. Moreover, foreign-born people are more likely than US-born people to start a company, according to Fairlie's 2012 study. And according to the Kauffman Foundation, about 44 percent of engineering and technology companies founded between 2006 and 2012 had at least one founder who was born abroad. Our health care system would benefit by way of important advances, new jobs, and more tax revenues from the efforts of highly educated people.

What Is the Total Cost of the Atlas Health Plan?

My plan will undoubtedly reduce the current level of national health expenditures, and consumers will save on the cost of insurance and the cost of health care. Nonetheless, it is difficult at best to separate and project over the long term the extremely complex and overlapping impacts of health system reforms. Moreover, in the context of cheaper medical care that will clearly result from these reforms, I have not included any of the other positive economic impacts, such as the anticipated rise in employee wages or job growth as a consequence of the reforms outlined in this plan. Given those limitations, I estimate the financial impacts from this plan over the first decade using reasonable approximations based on published literature and previous estimates of the JCT and the CBO, as indicated in Tables Q&A.1 and Q&A.2 below.

TABLE Q&A.1 Impact of Atlas Plan on Private Savings and Costs, Over Decade (approximations)

Specific Reform	Estimated Savings (Loss) over Decade	Reform Category (See Plan)
Remove penalties on uninsured people and employers	$210B*	Reform #1: Private insurance expansion
Remove excise tax on health insurance premiums	$87B*	Reform #1: Private insurance expansion
Premiums from shift to lower-cost, limited-mandate coverage[1]	$940B**	Reform #1: Private insurance expansion
Expanded HSA enrollment and limits[2]	$350B**	Reform #2: Universal liberalized HSAs
Transparency to consumers[3]	$880B**	Reform #2: Universal liberalized HSAs
Expanded utilization of wellness and lifestyle programs[4]	$120B**	Reform #2: Universal liberalized HSAs
Reduced income exclusion	($550B*)	Reform #3: Tax reforms
High-deductible option and new, expanded HSAs[5]	$400B**	Reform #4: Medicare modernization
Gradually phased-in increase in age of eligibility	($64B*)	Reform #4: Medicare modernization
High-deductible option and new, expanded HSAs[6]	$50B**	Reform #5: Medicaid overhaul
Repeal of taxes on devices and brand-name drugs	$196B*	Reform #6: Supply increases

(continued on next page)

TABLE Q&A.1. (continued)

Specific Reform	Estimated Savings (Loss) over Decade	Reform Category (See Plan)
Increased supply of retail clinics[7]	$20B**	Reform #6: Supply increases
Medical liability reforms[8]	$110B**	Reform #6: Supply increases

Overall Net Private Savings*:**
$2,749,000,000,000 (~$2.75T), over decade

[1] Estimated 5 percent savings per year from current projections on total private premiums paid, based on half of the 63 percent of privately insured who were not already in high-deductible plans switching, estimated 10 percent overall price drop in high-deductible plans from reduced mandates and more competition among insurers, and estimated 10 percent lower premiums for all existing and future high-deductible health plans extrapolating from one-half of other competition-induced health care price decreases. Data from US Department of Health/CDC/National Center for Health Statistics, June 2015 (see Table 10 in Health Insurance Coverage: Early Release of Estimates from the National Health Interview Survey, 2014), and CMS (see Exhibit 2 in S. P. Keehan et al., "National Health Expenditure Projections, 2014–24: Spending Growth Faster Than Recent Trends," *Health Affairs* 2015 [34]: 1407–17, http://content.healthaffairs.org/content/early/2015/07/15/hlthaff.2015.0600).

[2] Estimated from extrapolating extra savings from HSAs on expenditures with high-deductible plans of 5.5 percent to 14.1 percent (see Haviland, 2011); overall estimate of a 5 percent expected additional savings in all health expenditures for non–senior citizens because of widespread HSA enrollment.

[3] Estimated from transparency impact on reductions in spending for outpatient services assuming 19 percent reduction (see S-J Wu et al., "Price Transparency for MRIs Increased Use of Less Costly Providers and Triggered Provider Competition," *Health Affairs* 33 [2014]: 1391–98, http://content.healthaffairs.org/content/33/8/1391.abstract; and J. C. Robinson et al., "Reference-Based Benefit Design Changes Consumers' Choices and Employers' Payments for Ambulatory Surgery," *Health Affairs* 34 [2015]: 415–22, http://content.healthaffairs.org/content/34/3/415.abstract); projected outpatient spending in employer-sponsored insurance (see Haviland, 2011, and A. M. Haviland et al., "Growth of Consumer-Directed Health Plans to One-Half of All Employer-Sponsored Insurance Could Save $57 Billion Annually," *Health Affairs* 31, no. 5 [2012]: 1009–15, http://content.healthaffairs.org/content/31/5/1009.full).

[4] Estimated from impact of multiple wellness programs on health spending, based on $200/year/employee savings and 50 percent employee participation (see Health and Economic Implications of Worksite Wellness Programs, American Institute for Preventive Medicine, 2010; also Bureau of Labor Statistics).

[5] Estimated for new money into HSAs, reduced payments of premiums for supplemental insurance, rebates to enrollees choosing low-premium plans, and savings for out-of-pocket Medicare health expenses.

[6] Estimated for new money into HSAs and accumulated savings resulting from consumer incentives and high-deductible plans for nondisabled, non-senior-adult enrollees into Medicaid.

[7] Estimated from Parente, 2013, and others.

[8] Estimated to save 20 percent of total annual associated costs of medical liability (see M. M. Mello et al., "National Costs of the Medical Liability System," *Health Affairs* 29 [2010]: 1569–77).

Notes: *Approximations based on CBO/JCT estimates over one decade of implementation; **other amounts derived from the literature, using conservative estimates and given expected price transparency and increase in higher deductibles with HSAs (see footnotes); ***not including anticipated rise in wages to employees resulting from response to health reforms.

TABLE Q&A.2. Impact of Atlas Plan on Government Spending, Over Decade (approximations)

Specific Reform	Estimated Change over Decade	Reform Category (See Plan)
Eliminate ACA exchange subsidies	$822B* spending reduction	Reform #1: Private insurance expansion
Premium support with competitive bidding	$275B* spending reduction	Reform #4: Medicare modernization
Fixed federal grants to states, capped by CPI-U annual increases	$450B* spending reduction	Reform #5: Medicaid overhaul

Overall Government Spending Reduction:
$1,547,000,000,000 (-$1.5T) less, over decade

Note: *Approximations based on CBO/JCT estimates over one decade of implementation.

Notes

Chapter 1

1. S. P. Keehan et al., "National Health Expenditure Projections, 2014–24: Spending Growth Faster Than Recent Trends, *Health Affairs* 2015 (34): 1407–17, http://content.healthaffairs.org/content/early/2015/07/15/hlthaff.2015.0600.

2. Centers for Medicare and Medicaid Services, *Medicaid and CHIP: February 2015 Monthly Applications, Eligibility Determinations and Enrollment Report* (Baltimore, MD: Department of Health and Human Services, May 2015).

3. Centers for Medicare and Medicaid Services, Office of the Actuary, "2014 Annual Report of the Boards of Trustees of the Federal Hospital Insurance and Federal Supplementary Medical Insurance Trust Funds," July 2014, https://www.cms.gov/research-statistics-data-and-systems/statistics-trends-and-reports/reportstrustfunds/downloads/tr2014.pdf.

4. Ibid.

5. National Research Council and National Academy of Public Administration, *Choosing the Nation's Fiscal Future* (Washington, DC: National Academy of Sciences, 2011).

6. Soeren Mattke, "Health Care Quality Indicators Project: Initial Indicators Report" (OECD Health Working Paper 22, Organisation for Economic Co-operation and Development, Paris, France, 2006); Sandra Garcia Armesto et al., "Health Care Quality Indicators Project 2006: Data Collection Update Report" (OECD Health Working Paper 29, Organisation for Economic Co-operation and Development, Paris, France, 2007); M. J. Quinn, "Cancer Trends in the United States: A View from Europe, *Journal of the National Cancer Institute* 95 (2003): 1258–61; G. Gatta et al., "Toward a Comparison of Survival in American and European Cancer Patients," *Cancer* 89 (2000): 899; L. Ciccolallo et al., "Survival Differences between European and US Patients with Colorectal Cancer: Role of Stage at Diagnosis and Surgery," *Gut* 54 (2005): 268–73; D. H. Howard et al., "Cancer Screening and Age in the United States and Europe," *Health Affairs* 28 (2009): 1838–47; June O'Neill and Dave M. O'Neill, "Health Status, Health Care and Inequality: Canada vs. the U.S." (NBER Working Paper 13429, National Bureau of Economic Research, Cambridge, MA, September 2007).

7. M. A. Richards, "The Size of the Prize for Earlier Diagnosis of Cancer in England," *British Journal of Cancer* 101, suppl 2 (2009): S125–29; E. R. Salomaa et al., "Delays in the Diagnosis and Treatment of Lung Cancer," *Chest* 128 (2005): 2282–88; "Public Patients Face Up to Five-Year Wait to See a Specialist," *Independent*, March 25, 2011, http://www.independent.ie/health/latest-news/public -patients-face-up-to-fiveyear-wait-to-see-a-specialist-2594298.html; Jeremy Hurst and Luigi Siciliani, "Tackling Excessive Waiting Times for Elective Surgery: A Comparison of Policies in Twelve OECD Countries" (OECD Health Working Paper 6, Organisation for Economic Co-operation and Development, Paris, France, 2003); B. Barua and F. Fathers, "Waiting Your Turn: Wait Times for Health Care in Canada, 2014 Report," Fraser Institute, https://www .fraserinstitute.org/sites/default/files/waiting-your-turn-2014.pdf; Merritt Hawkins, "Physician Appointment Wait Times and Medicaid and Medicare Acceptance Rates, 2014 Annual Survey," http://www.merritthawkins.com /uploadedFiles/MerrittHawkins/Surveys/mha2014waitsurvPDF.pdf; C. Schoen et al., "The Commonwealth Fund 2010 International Health Policy Survey in Eleven Countries," November 2010, http://www.commonwealthfund.org/~ /media/files/publications/chartbook/2010/pdf_2010_ihp_survey_chartpack _full_12022010.pdf.

8. K. Wolf-Maier et al., "Hypertension Treatment and Control in Five European Countries, Canada, and the United States," *Hypertension* 43 (2004): 10–17; K. E. Thorpe et al., "Differences in Disease Prevalence as a Source of the U.S.-European Health Care Spending Gap," *Health Affairs* 26 (2007): 678–86; Eileen M. Crimmins et al., "Are International Differences in Health Similar to International Differences in Life Expectancy?" in *International Differences in Mortality at Older Ages: Dimensions and Sources*, ed. E. M. Crimmins et al. (Washington, DC: The National Academies Press), tables 3.4 and 3.6; O'Neill and O'Neill, "Health Status, Health Care and Inequality."

9. Richards, "The Size of the Prize for Earlier Diagnosis of Cancer in England"; Salomaa, "Delays in the Diagnosis and Treatment of Lung Cancer"; "Public Patients Face Up to Five-Year Wait," *Independent*; Hurst and Siciliani, "Tackling Excessive Waiting Times"; Barua and Fathers, "Waiting Your Turn"; Scott W. Atlas, "Evaluating Access to America's Medical Care," in *In Excellent Health: Setting the Record Straight on America's Health Care* (Stanford, CA: Hoover Press, 2011).

10. See, for example, B. Barua et al., "The Effect of Wait Times on Mortality in Canada," Fraser Institute, May 2014, https://www.fraserinstitute.org/sites /default/files/effect-of-wait-times-on-mortality-in-canada.pdf; M. Snider et al., "Waiting Times and Patient Perspectives for Total Hip and Knee Arthroplasty in Rural and Urban Ontario," *Canadian Journal of Surgery* 48 (2005): 355–60; Hurst and Siciliani, "Tackling Excessive Waiting Times"; J. Ethier et al., "Vascular Access Use and Outcomes: An International Perspective from the Dialysis Outcomes and Practice Patterns Study," *Nephrology Dialysis Transplantation*

23 (2008): 3219–26; L. Moon et al., "Stroke Care in OECD Countries: A Comparison of Treatment, Costs, and Outcomes in 17 Countries (Annex)" (OECD Health Working Papers 5, Organisation for Economic Co-operation and Development, Paris, France, 2003), table A2.6; R. J. Blendon et al., "Confronting Competing Demands to Improve Quality: A Five-Country Hospital Survey," *Health Affairs* 23 (2004): 119–35; Agency for Healthcare Research and Quality, "Cardiac Catheterization in Freestanding Clinics," Technology Assessment, September 7, 2005, https://www.cms.gov/Medicare/Coverage/DeterminationProcess/downloads/id28TA.pdf; J. Z. Ayanian and T. J. Quinn, "Quality of Care for Coronary Heart Disease in Two Countries," *Health Affairs* 20 (2001): 55–67.

11. See, for example, M. O. Baerlocher, "Canada's Slow Adoption of New Technologies Adds Burden to Health Care System," *Canadian Medical Association Journal* 176 (2007): 616.

12. B. Jonsson and N. Wilking, "Market Uptake of New Oncology Drugs," *Annals of Oncology* 18, suppl 3 (2007): iii2–iii7, doi:10.1093/annonc/mdm099; European Federation of Pharmaceutical Industries and Associations, "The Pharmaceutical Industry in Figures, Key Data: 2011 Update," http://www.efpia.eu/content/default.asp?PageID=559&DocID=11586; Peter Mitchell, "Price Controls Seen as Key to Europe's Drug Innovation Lag," *Nature Reviews Drug Discovery* 6 (2007): 257–58, doi:10.1038/nrd2293; Tufts Center for the Study of Drug Development, "While Total Approvals Decline, U.S. Is Preferred Market for First Launch, *Impact Report* 10 (November/December 2008), http://csdd.tufts.edu/files/uploads/novdeco8summary.pdf.

13. For a detailed review, see Atlas, "Evaluating Access to America's Medical Care," 159–210.

14. For a detailed review, see Atlas, "Measuring Medical Care Quality in the United States," 97–158.

15. See, for example, A. Verdecchia et al., "Recent Cancer Survival in Europe: A 2000–02 Period Analysis of EUROCARE-4 Data," *Lancet Oncology* 8 (2007): 784–96; Concord Working Group, "Cancer Survival in Five Continents: A Worldwide Population-Based Study," *Lancet Oncology* 9, no. 8 (2008): 730–56.

16. See, for example, F. Levi et al., "Trends in Mortality from Cardiovascular and Cerebrovascular Diseases in Europe and Other Areas of the World, *Heart* 88 (2002): 119–24; P. Kaul et al., Long-Term Mortality of Patients with Acute Myocardial Infarction in the United States and Canada, *Circulation* 110 (2004): 1754–60; Melissa L. Martinson et al., "Health across the Life Span in the United States and England," *American Journal of Epidemiology*, March 9, 2011, doi: 10.1093/aje/kwq325; J. Z. Ayanian and T. J. Quinn, "Quality of Care for Coronary Heart Disease in Two Countries," *Health Affairs* 20 (2001): 55–67; H. C. Wijeysundera et al., "Association of Temporal Trends in Risk Factors and Treatment Uptake with Coronary Heart Disease Mortality, 1994–2005," *Journal*

of the American Medical Association 303 (2010): 1841–47; Thorpe et al., "Differences in Disease Prevalence."

17. See, for example, Wolf-Maier et al., "Hypertension Treatment and Control"; Y. R. Wang et al., "Outpatient Hypertension Treatment, Treatment Intensification, and Control in Western Europe and the United States," *Archives of Internal Medicine* 167 (2007): 141–47; E. Gakidou et al., "Management of Diabetes and Associated Cardiovascular Risk Factors in Seven Countries: A Comparison of Data from National Health Examination Surveys," *Bulletin of the World Health Organization* 89 (2011): 172–83.

18. See, for example, C. Almeida et al., "Methodological Concerns and Recommendations on Policy Consequences of the *World Health Report 2000*," *Lancet* 357 (2001): 1692; P. Musgrove, "Judging Health Systems: Reflections on WHO's Methods," *Lancet* 361 (2003): 1817–20; E. Ollila and M. Koivusalo, "The *World Health Report 2000*: The World Health Organization Health Policy Steering Off-Course: Changed Values, Poor Evidence, and Lack of Accountability," *International Journal of Health Services* 32 (2002): 503–14; Scott W. Atlas, "The WHO Ranking of Health Systems Redux: A Critical Appraisal," in *In Excellent Health: Setting the Record Straight on America's Health Care* (Stanford, CA: Hoover Press, 2011), 1–18.

19. Congressional Budget Office, "Insurance Coverage Provisions of the Affordable Care Act—CBO's March 2015 Baseline," March 2015, https://www.cbo.gov/sites/default/files/cbofiles/attachments/43900-2015-03-ACAtables.pdf.

20. Edmund F. Haislmaier and Drew Gonshorowski, "Q3 2014 Health Insurance Enrollment: Employer Coverage Continues to Decline, Medicaid Keeps Growing" (Heritage Foundation Backgrounder 2988, January 29, 2015), http://www.heritage.org/research/reports/2015/01/q3-2014-health-insurance-enrollment-employer-coverage-continues-to-decline-medicaid-keeps-growing.

21. Centers for Medicare and Medicaid Services, "National Health Expenditure Projections, 2012–2022," https://www.cms.gov/research-statistics-data-and-systems/statistics-trends-and-reports/nationalhealthexpenddata/downloads/proj2012.pdf.

Chapter 2

1. Centers for Studying Health System Change, "CTS Physician Surveys and the HSC 2008 Health Tracking Physician Survey," http://www.hschange.com/index.cgi?data=04.

2. Merritt Hawkins, "Physician Appointment Wait Times and Medicaid and Medicare Acceptance Rates, 2014 Annual Survey," http://www.merritthawkins.com/uploadedFiles/MerrittHawkins/Surveys/mha2014waitsurvPDF.pdf.

3. Department of Health and Human Services, "Access to Care: Provider Availability in Medicaid Managed Care," Report OEI-02-13-00670 (December 2014), http://oig.hhs.gov/oei/reports/oei-02-13-00670.pdf.

4. Medicare Payment Advisory Commission, *Report to the Congress: Medicare Payment Policy*. Washington, DC: MedPAC, March 2009.

5. Physicians Foundation, "2014 Survey of America's Physicians: Practice Patterns and Perspectives, http://www.physiciansfoundation.org/uploads/default /2014_Physicians_Foundation_Biennial_Physician_Survey_Report.pdf.

6. Physicians Foundation, "2012 Survey of America's Physicians: Practice Patterns and Perspectives," http://www.physiciansfoundation.org/uploads/default /Physicians_Foundation_2012_Biennial_Survey.pdf.

7. See, for example, Michael A. Gaglia, "Effect of Insurance Type on Adverse Cardiac Events after Percutaneous Coronary Intervention," *American Journal of Cardiology* 107 (2011): 675–80; D. J. LaPar et al., "Primary Payer Status Affects Mortality for Major Surgical Operations," *Annals of Surgery* 252 (2010): 544–51; J. Kwok et al., "The Impact of Health Insurance Status on the Survival of Patients with Head and Neck Cancer," *Cancer* 116 (2010): 476–85; R. R. Kelz et al., "Morbidity and Mortality of Colorectal Carcinoma Differs by Insurance Status," *Cancer* 101 (2004): 2187–94; J. G. Allen et al., "Insurance Status Is an Independent Predictor of Long-Term Survival after Lung Transplantation in the United States," *Journal of Heart and Lung Transplantation* 30 (2011): 45–53.

8. Congressional Budget Office, "Insurance Coverage Provisions of the Affordable Care Act—CBO's January 2015 Baseline," https://www.cbo.gov/sites /default/files/cbofiles/attachments/43900-2015-01-ACAtables.pdf.

9. W. Fox and J. Pickering, "Hospital and Physician Cost Shift: Payment Level Comparison of Medicare, Medicaid, and Commercial Payers," *Milliman Client Report*, December 2008, http://www.milliman.com/expertise/healthcare /publications/rr/pdfs/hospital-physician-cost-shift-RR12-01-08.pdf.

10. American Hospital Association and Avalere Health, *Trendwatch Chartbook 2014: Trends Affecting Hospitals and Health Systems* (Washington, DC: American Hospital Association, 2014), http://www.aha.org/research/reports/tw /chartbook/2014/14chartbook.pdf.

11. Alyene Senger, "Measuring Choice and Competition in the Exchanges: Still Worse Than before the ACA" (Heritage Foundation Issue Brief 4324 on Health Care, December 22, 2014), http://www.heritage.org/research/reports /2014/12/measuring-choice-and-competition-in-the-exchanges-still-worse -than-before-the-aca.

12. E. Coe et al., "Hospital Networks: Configurations on the Exchanges and Their Impact on Premiums," McKinsey Center for U.S. Health System Reform (December 2013), http://healthcare.mckinsey.com/hospital-networks -configurations-exchanges-and-their-impact-premiums.

13. Avalere Health, "Access to Comprehensive Stroke Centers and Specialty Physicians in Exchange Plans," September 2014, http://www.heart.org/idc/groups /public/@wcm/@adv/documents/downloadable/ucm_468318.pdf.

14. Avalere Health, "Exchange Plans Include 34 Percent Fewer Providers Than the Average for Commercial Plans," June 2015, http://avalere.com/expertise /managed-care/insights/exchange-plans-include-34-percent-fewer-providers -than-the-average-for-comm.

15. Kaiser Family Foundation, "Employee Health Benefits Annual Surveys, 2007–2014," http://kff.org/health-costs/report/employer-health-benefits-annual -survey-archives.

16. A. Haviland et al., "Do 'Consumer-Directed' Health Plans Bend the Cost Curve over Time? (NBER Working Paper 21031, National Bureau of Economic Research, Cambridge, MA, March 2015), http://www.nber.org/papers/w21031.

17. A. Haviland et al., "How Do Consumer-Directed Health Plans Affect Vulnerable Populations?" *Forum for Health Economics and Policy* 14, no. 2 (2011): 1–12, online, doi: 10.2202/1558-9544.1248.

18. A. M. Haviland et al., "The Effects of Consumer-Directed Health Plans on Episodes of Health Care," *Forum for Health Economics and Policy* 14, no. 2 (2011): 1–27, http://www.rand.org/pubs/external_publications/EP201100208 .html.

19. S-J Wu et al., "Price Transparency for MRIs Increased Use of Less Costly Providers and Triggered Provider Competition," *Health Affairs* 33 (2014): 1391–98, http://content.healthaffairs.org/content/33/8/1391.abstract.

20. J. C. Robinson et al., "Reference-Based Benefit Design Changes Consumers' Choices and Employers' Payments for Ambulatory Surgery," *Health Affairs* 34 (2015): 415–22, http://content.healthaffairs.org/content/34/3/415.abstract.

21. Based on my analysis of the Kaiser Family Foundation's employer health benefits annual survey data, 2006–2014; see Kaiser Family Foundation, http:// kff.org/health-costs/report/employer-health-benefits-annual-survey-archives/

22. Edmund F. Haislmaier and Drew Gonshorowski, "Responding to *King v. Burwell*: Congress's First Step Should Be to Remove Costly Mandates Driving Up Premiums" (Heritage Foundation Issue Brief 4400, May 2015), http://www .heritage.org/research/reports/2015/05/responding-to-king-v-burwell-congresss -first-step-should-be-to-remove-costly-mandates-driving-up-premiums.

23. Council for Affordable Health Insurance, "Health Insurance Mandates in the States 2012," http://www.cahi.org/cahi_contents/resources/pdf /Mandatesinthestates2012Execsumm.pdf.

24. James T. O'Connor, "Comprehensive Assessment of ACA Factors That Will Affect Individual Market Premiums in 2014," *Milliman Reports*, April 25, 2013, http://ahip.org/MillimanReportACA2013/.

25. American Academy of Actuaries, "Drivers of 2016 Health Insurance Premium Changes," Issue Brief, August 2015, http://actuary.org/files/Drivers_2016 _Premiums_080515.pdf.

26. Chris Carlson, "Annual Tax on Insurers Allocated by State," Oliver Wyman Report, November 2012, http://www.ahip.org/WymanReportNov2012/.

27. B. E. Garrett et al., "Cigarette Smoking: United States, 1965–2008," *Morbidity and Mortality Weekly Report (MMWR)*, Centers for Disease Control and Prevention 60 (January 14, 2011): 109–13.

28. D. Withrow and D. A. Alter, "The Economic Burden of Obesity Worldwide: A Systematic Review of the Direct Costs of Obesity," *Obesity Reviews* 12 (2011): 131–41.

29. R. A. Hammond and R. Levine, "The Economic Impact of Obesity in the United States," *Diabetes, Metabolic Syndrome and Obesity: Targets and Therapy* 3 (2010): 285–95.

30. E. A. Finkelstein et al., "Obesity and Severe Obesity Forecasts through 2030," *American Journal of Preventive Medicine* 42, no. 6 (2012): 563–70 (italics added for emphasis).

31. See, for example, J. Wellington, press release, Doermer School of Business and Management Sciences, Indiana University—Purdue University Fort Wayne, 2007; M. Endres et al., "Primary Prevention of Stroke: Blood Pressure, Lipids, and Heart Failure," *European Heart Journal* 32 (2011): 545–55.

32. W. N. Burton et al., "The Economic Costs Associated with Body Mass Index in a Workplace," *Journal of Occupational and Environmental Medicine* 40 (1998): 786–92.

33. Finkelstein et al., "Obesity and Severe Obesity Forecasts," 563–70.

34. "Smoking Status and Body Mass Index Relative to Average Individual Health Insurance Premiums," *eHealth* (2011), http://news.ehealthinsurance.com /_ir/68/20125/Smoking_Status_BMI_and_Individual_Health_Insurance _Premiums.pdf.

Chapter 3

1. Devenir Research, "2015 Midyear HSA Market Statistics and Trends," August 11, 2015, http://www.devenir.com/research/2015-midyear-devenir-hsa -research-report/.

2. A. M. Haviland et al., "The Effects of Consumer-Directed Health Plans on Episodes of Health Care," *Forum for Health Economics and Policy* 14, no. 2 (2011): 1–27, http://www.rand.org/pubs/external_publications/EP201100208 .html.

3. A. M. Haviland et al., "Growth of Consumer-Directed Health Plans to One-Half of All Employer-Sponsored Insurance Could Save $57 Billion Annually," *Health Affairs* 31, no. 5 (2012): 1009–15, http://content.healthaffairs.org /content/31/5/1009.full.

4. National Business Group on Health, "Taking Action to Improve Employee Health: Results from the Sixth Annual Employer-Sponsored Health and

Well-being Survey," March 25, 2015, https://www.businessgrouphealth.org
/pub/29d50202-782b-cb6e-2763-a29a9426f589.

5. Kaiser Foundation and Heath Research and Educational Trust, "2014
Employer Health Benefits Survey, Section 12: Wellness Programs and Risk
Assessments," September 2014, http://kff.org/report-section/ehbs-2014-section
-twelve-wellness-programs-and-health-risk-assessments/.

6. L. L. Berry et al., "What's the Hard Return on Employee Wellness
Programs?" *Harvard Business Review*, December 2010, https://hbr.org/2010/12
/whats-the-hard-return-on-employee-wellness-programs.

7. K. Baicker et al., "Workplace Wellness Programs Can Generate Savings,"
Health Affairs 29 (2010): 304–11.

Chapter 4

1. Beth Stevens, "Blurring the Boundaries: How the Federal Government Has
Influenced Welfare Benefits in the Private Sector," in *The Politics of Social Policy in the United States*, ed. Margaret Weir, Ann Shola Orloff, and Theda Skocpol
(Princeton, NJ: Princeton University Press, 1988).

2. Paul Starr, *The Social Transformation of American Medicine* (New York:
Basic Books, 1982).

3. Robert B. Helms, "Tax Policy and the History of the Health Insurance
Industry" (paper presented at the Taxes and Health Insurance: Analysis and
Policy Conference, Brookings Institution, February 29, 2008), http://www
.taxpolicycenter.org/tpccontent/healthconference_helms.pdf.

4. Congressional Budget Office, "Options for Reducing the Deficit: 2014 to
2023," November 2013, http://www.cbo.gov/sites/default/files/cbofiles/attachments
/44715-OptionsForReducingDeficit-3.pdf; see especially "Health Revenues—
Option 15," p. 243.

5. S. Lowry, "Itemized Tax Deductions for Individuals: Data Analysis," Congressional Research Service, February 2014, http://www.fas.org/sgp/crs/misc
/R43012.pdf.

6. Congressional Budget Office, "Options for Reducing the Deficit: 2014 to
2023."

7. Jonathan Gruber, "The Tax Exclusion for Employer-Sponsored Health
Insurance," *National Tax Journal* 64, no. 2, pt. 2 (June 2011): 511–30.

8. Jonathan Gruber and Brigitte Madrian, "Health Insurance, Labor Supply,
and Job Mobility: A Critical Review of the Literature," in *Health Policy and the
Uninsured*, ed. Catherine McLaughlin (Washington, DC: Urban Institute Press,
2004), 97–108.

9. M. Feldstein and B. Friedman, "Tax Subsidies, the Rational Demand for
Insurance and the Health Care Crisis," *Journal of Public Economics* (1977):
155–78.

10. See, for example, A. Finkelstein, "The Aggregate Effects of Health Insurance: Evidence from the Introduction of Medicare," *Quarterly Journal of Economics* 122 (2007): 1–37.

11. Unless compensated in significantly lower overall tax rates and higher after-tax income. I make the assumption that comprehensive tax reform into a broad-based, low-tax-rate system will not likely occur.

12. JCT/CBO estimates based on limits at $6,420 for individuals and $15,620 for families; see Congressional Budget Office, "Options for Reducing the Deficit: 2014 to 2023."

13. Congressional Budget Office, "Options for Reducing the Deficit: 2014 to 2023."

14. Gruber, "Tax Exclusion for Employer-Sponsored Health Insurance."

15. L. Clemans-Cope et al., "Limiting the Tax Exclusion of Employer-Sponsored Health Insurance Premiums: Revenue Potential and Distributional Consequences," RWJ Foundation and the Urban Institute, May 2013, http://www.urban.org/sites/default/files/alfresco/publication-pdfs/412816-Limiting-the-Tax-Exclusion-of-Employer-Sponsored-Health-Insurance-Premiums-Revenue-Potential-and-Distributional-Consequences.PDF.

Chapter 5

1. C. Twight, "Medicare's Origin: The Economics and Politics of Dependency," *Cato Journal* 16, no. 3 (Winter 1997): 309–38.

2. US Government Accountability Office, "High-Risk Series: An Update," February 2015, 359, http://www.gao.gov/assets/670/668415.pdf.

3. Actuarial data from HealthView using historical claim data and projections, June 2011.

4. J. M. Ortman et al., "An Aging Nation: The Older Population in the United States: Population Estimates and Projection," US Census Bureau Current Population Reports, no. P25-1140, May 2014, https://www.census.gov/prod/2014pubs/p25-1140.pdf.

5. Howard Dean, "The Affordable Care Acts Rate-Setting Won't Work, *Wall Street Journal*, July 28, 2013.

6. American Medical Association, "National Health Insurer Report Card, 2013," https://www.trizetto.com/WorkArea/DownloadAsset.aspx?id=6385.

7. Physicians Foundation, "2014 Survey of America's Physicians: Practice Patterns and Perspectives," http://www.physiciansfoundation.org/uploads/default/2014_Physicians_Foundation_Biennial_Physician_Survey_Report.pdf.

8. G. Jacobson et al., "Medigap Reform: Setting the Context for Understanding Recent Proposals," Henry J. Kaiser Family Foundation, January 2014, http://kff.org/medicare/issue-brief/medigap-reform-setting-the-context/.

9. Henry J. Kaiser Family Foundation, "Medicare Advantage: Fact Sheet," June 2015, http://files.kff.org/attachment/fact-sheet-medicare-advantage.

10. See Walton Francis, *Putting Medicare Consumers in Charge: Lessons from the FEHBP* (Washington, DC: AEI Press, 2009).

11. See ibid.

12. See Robert E. Moffit, "Saving the American Dream: Comparing Medicare Reforms Plans" (Heritage Foundation Backgrounder 2675, April 4, 2012), http://www.heritage.org/research/reports/2012/04/saving-the-american-dream-comparing-medicare-reform-plans.

13. Congressional Budget Office, "Options for Reducing the Deficit: 2014 to 2023," November 2013, http://www.cbo.gov/sites/default/files/cbofiles/attachments/44715-OptionsForReducingDeficit-3.pdf.

14. Rebecca Riffkin, "Average U.S. Retirement Age Rises to 62," Gallup, April 2014, http://www.gallup.com/poll/168707/average-retirement-age-rises.aspx.

15. Congressional Budget Office, "Options for Reducing the Deficit: 2014 to 2023," November 2013, http://www.cbo.gov/sites/default/files/cbofiles/attachments/44715-OptionsForReducingDeficit-3.pdf; see especially "Health Revenues—Option 15," p. 243.

Chapter 6

1. S. P. Keehan et al., "National Health Expenditure Projections, 2014–24: Spending Growth Faster Than Recent Trends," *Health Affairs* 34 (2015): 1407–17, http://content.healthaffairs.org/content/early/2015/07/15/hlthaff.2015.0600.

2. Congressional Research Service, "Questions about the ACA Medicaid Expansion," Memorandum, January 30, 2015, https://www.heartland.org/sites/default/files/crs_memo_-_questions_about_the_aca_medicaid_expansion_-_jan_2015.pdf.

Chapter 7

1. J. S. Ashwood et al., "Trends in Retail Clinic Use among the Commercially Insured," *American Journal of Managed Care* 17, no. 11 (2011): e443–e448.

2. A. Mehrotra et al., "The Costs and Quality of Care for Three Common Illnesses at Retail Clinics as Compared to Other Medical Settings," *Annals of Internal Medicine* 151, no. 5 (2009): 321–28.

3. R. M. Weinick et al., "Policy Implications of the Use of Retail Clinics," Rand Health Technical Report, 2010, http://www.rand.org/content/dam/rand/pubs/technical_reports/2010/RAND_TR810.pdf.

4. Accenture, "Retail Medical Clinics Will Double between 2012 and 2015 and Save $800 Million per Year," June 2013, https://www.accenture.com

/_acnmedia/Accenture/Conversion-Assets/DotCom/Documents/Global/PDF
/Dualpub_21/Accenture-Retail-Medical-Clinics-From-Foe-to-Friend.pdf.

5. Ashwood et al., "Trends in Retail Clinic Use."

6. R. Rudavsky et al., "The Geographic Distribution, Ownership, Prices, and Scope of Practice at Retail Clinics," *Annals of Internal Medicine* 151 (2009): 315–20.

7. Committee on the Robert Wood Foundation Initiative on the Future of Nursing, *The Future of Nursing: Leading Change, Advancing Health* (Washington, DC: National Academies Press, 2011), http://www.nap.edu/catalog/12956/the-future-of-nursing-leading-change-advancing-health.

8. Association of American Medical Colleges, "The Complexities of Physician Supply and Demand: Projections through 2025," Report of the Center for Workforce Studies, 2008, https://members.aamc.org/eweb/upload/The%20Complexities%20of%20Physician%20Supply.pdf.

9. Centers for Disease Control and Prevention/National Center for Health Statistics, *Population Aging and the Use of Office-based Physician Services*, NCHS Data Brief No. 41, August 2010; National Ambulatory Medical Care Survey, 1978 and 2008; see http://www.cdc.gov/nchs/data/databriefs/db41.PDF.

10. M. M. Mello et al., "National Costs of the Medical Liability System," *Health Affairs* 29 (2010): 1569–77.

11. "2014 Global R&D Funding Forecast," Battelle and *R&D Magazine*, https://www.battelle.org/docs/tpp/2014_global_rd_funding_forecast.pdf.

12. M. J. Lamberti and K. Getz, Tufts Center for the Study of Drug Development, May 2015; F. Pammolli et al., "The Productivity Crisis in Pharmaceutical R&D," *Nature Reviews Drug Discovery* 10 (2011): 428–38.

13. J. Makower et al., "FDA Impact on US Medical Technology Innovation," November 2010, http://eucomed.org/uploads/Press%20Releases/FDA%20impact%20on%20U.S.%20Medical%20Technology%20Innovation.pdf.

14. PricewaterhouseCooper, "Medical Technology Innovation Scorecard," 2011, http://pwchealth.com/cgi-local/hregister.cgi/reg/innovation-scorecard.pdf.

15. Vivek Wadhwa, *The Immigrant Exodus: Why America Is Losing the Global Race to Capture Entrepreneurial Talent* (Philadelphia: Wharton Digital Press, 2012).

Conclusion

1. Scott W. Atlas, "The Surprising International Consensus on Healthcare," *Defining Ideas*, June 19, 2014, http://www.hoover.org/research/surprising-international-consensus-healthcare; Scott W. Atlas, ed., *Reforming America's Health Care System: The Flawed Vision of ObamaCare* (Stanford, CA: Hoover

Press, 2010); Scott W. Atlas, *In Excellent Health: Setting the Record Straight on America's Health Care* (Stanford, CA: Hoover Press, 2011).

2. CEA Insurers of Europe, "Private Medical Insurance in the European Union, 2011," http://docplayer.net/1002288-Cea-insurers-of-europe-private -medical-insurance-in-the-european-union.html.

3. For example, in the United Kingdom alone, the total number of patients on the waiting list for diagnosis or start of treatment reached 3.4 million in May 2015, the highest since 2008, including the 11.8 percent of hospitalized patients whose wait exceeded eighteen weeks; 18 percent of UK cancer patients referred for "urgent treatment" were forced to wait more than two full months for initiation of treatment (see Kings Fund, "How Is the NHS Performing?, *NHS Quarterly Monitoring Report*, July 2015, http://qmr.kingsfund.org.uk/2015/16/.)

4. NHS Choices, "The NHS in England," http://www.nhs.uk/NHSEngland /thenhs/about/Pages/overview.aspx.

5. LaingBuisson, "Health Cover UK Market Report," 12th ed., 2015, https:// www.laingbuisson.co.uk/Portals/1/MarketReports/Documents/Health_Cover _12ed_Bro_WEB.pdf.

6. Insurance Sweden, "Insurance in Sweden: Statistics 2013," 2013, http:// www.svenskforsakring.se/PageFiles/6717/SF_Statistikbroschyr_2013_eng.pdf ?epslanguage=sv.

7. Rasmussen survey, June 2015.

8. Rasmussen survey, September 25–27, 2015.

About the Author

Scott W. Atlas, MD, is the David and Joan Traitel Senior Fellow at Stanford University's Hoover Institution and a member of Hoover Institution's Working Group on Health Care Policy. He investigates the impact of government and the private sector on access, quality, pricing, and innovation in health care, and he is a frequent policy adviser to government leaders in those areas. Dr. Atlas's most recent books include *Reforming America's Health Care System* (Hoover Institution Press, 2010) and *In Excellent Health: Setting the Record Straight on America's Health Care System* (Hoover Institution Press, 2011). Dr. Atlas has been interviewed by or has published in a variety of media, including BBC Radio, the PBS *NewsHour*, the *Wall Street Journal*, *Forbes Magazine*, CNN, *USA Today*, Fox News, London's *Financial Times*, Brazil's *Correio Braziliense*, Italy's *Corriere della Sera*, and Argentina's *Diario La Nacion*. Dr. Atlas also advises entrepreneurs and companies in the life sciences, medical technology, and health information technology sectors.

Dr. Atlas is also the editor of the leading textbook in the field, *Magnetic Resonance Imaging of the Brain and Spine*, being published in its fifth edition and previously translated from English into Mandarin, Spanish, and Portuguese. He has been an editor, an associate editor, and a member of the editorial and scientific boards of many journals as well as national and international scientific societies during the past three decades and has written more than 120 scientific publications in leading journals. As professor and chief of neuroradiology at Stanford University Medical Center from 1998 until 2012 and during his prior academic positions, Dr. Atlas trained more than one hundred neuroradiology fellows, many of whom are now leaders in the field throughout the world.

Dr. Atlas received a BS degree in biology from the University of Illinois in Urbana-Champaign and an MD degree from the University of Chicago School of Medicine.

Index

access, 7–8
  ACA limits to health care, 1, 15–16,
    40, 41, 48, 61, 75
  HSAs and health care, 27
  Medicare and Medicaid reforms
    and, 44–45, 51, 83, 84, 86, 88
  private insurance and health care,
    11, 13, 14, 93
  retail clinics and health care,
    53–54
  to specialists, 15, 51, 53, 87
  two-tiered, 42
Affordable Care Act (ACA), 79
  access to health care under, 1,
    15–16, 40, 41, 48, 61, 75
  "Cadillac tax" under, 35–36, 81
  consolidation under, 1, 11, 15,
    74–75
  devices under, 43, 56–57, 58
  "guarantee issue" under, 71–72, 88
  HDHPs before and after, 19f, 20f, 21f
  insurance mandates and
    compliance, 20–21, 27, 67–68
  low-income earners impacted by,
    62
  market-based competition
    impacted by, 15, 73
  Medicaid enrollment under, 10–11,
    48
  pharmaceutical companies
    impacted by, 1, 11, 74
  private insurance impacted by,
    14–16, 18, 20–21, 20f, 21f, 67
  senior citizens under, 40–41

threat to innovation of, 1–2, 15–16,
  56–57, 58
US system prior to, 7–8, 65, 66
wellness incentives restricted by,
  29–30. *See also* Medicaid;
  Medicare; tax treatment of
  health spending
age
  elimination of premiums based on,
    13, 21
  expenditures per capita by, 40f
  Medicare reform and eligibility,
    46, 77, 88–89, 97f. *See also* life
    expectancy; senior citizens
aging, 1, 5–6, 10–11

beneficiaries, 87, 90, 91, 93, 94
body mass index (BMI), 7f, 23

"Cadillac tax," 35–36, 81
cancer treatment, 8, 9f, 57f, 59f, 89
CBO. *See* Congressional Budget
  Office
Centers for Medicare and Medicaid
  Services (CMS), 10, 14, 39, 86
clinics, retail. *See* retail clinics
competition. *See* market-based
  competition
Congressional Budget Office (CBO),
  97, 98, 99f
  private insurance projections by,
    14–15
  on tax treatment of health
    spending, 20–21, 32, 34, 35

115